Better partnership working

PARTNERSHIP WORKING IN HEALTH AND SOCIAL CARE

Better partnership working

Series editors: Jon Glasby and Helen Dickinson

About the authors

Jon Glasby is Professor of Health and Social Care at the Health Services Management Centre, University of Birmingham. He is also Director of Academic Programmes across the wider School of Public Policy. As a qualified social worker in an NHS setting, he leads a national programme of work to support the integration of adult health and social care.

Helen Dickinson is a researcher at the Health Services Management Centre, University of Birmingham, with an interest in evaluating the outcomes of health and social care partnerships. Recent research and consultancy work include producing research-based but accessible discussion papers for funders such as the Wanless Review of the funding of adult social care, the NHS Institute and the Care Services Improvement Partnership.

PARTNERSHIP WORKING IN HEALTH AND SOCIAL CARE

Jon Glasby and Helen Dickinson

in association with

COMMUNITYcare

First published in Great Britain in 2008 by

The Policy Press
University of Bristol
Fourth Floor, Beacon House
Queen's Road
Bristol BS8 1QU

Tel +44 (0)117 331 4054
Fax +44 (0)117 331 4093
e-mail tpp-info@bristol.ac.uk
www.policypress.org.uk

© Jon Glasby and Helen Dickinson 2008

British Library Cataloguing in Publication Data
A catalogue record for this book is available from the British Library

Library of Congress Cataloging-in-Publication Data
A catalog record for this book has been requested

ISBN 978 1 84742 016 9 paperback

Cover design by In-text Design, Bristol.
Printed and bound in Great Britain by MPG Books, Bodmin.

Contents

List of tables, figures and boxes

Tables

Figures

Boxes

—

LIST OF TABLES, FIGURES AND BOXES

Acknowledgements

The authors would like to thank The Policy Press and *Community Care*. In particular, they are grateful to the contributors to subsequent books in this series, as well as to the peer reviewers who acted as critical friends while each book was being written and edited.

The authors' thanks also go to the various people who have contributed personal opinions and experiences to this book, and who have allowed them to reproduce their material. Particular thanks go to Rob Greig for permission to reproduce Figures 3.1 and 3.2, to Chris Skelcher and colleagues for permission to reproduce their Governance Assessment Tool in Box 3.5 and a summary of different theoretical approaches to partnership working in Table 4.3, to the Integrated Care Network for permission to reproduce Boxes 4.3–4.6 and to Annette Hastings for permission to reproduce Tables 4.1 and 4.2.

Any opinions (and indeed errors) in the book are those of the authors.

List of abbreviations

Health and social care use a large number of abbreviations and acronyms. Some of the more popular terms used in this book are set out below:

A&E	Accident and Emergency
AHP	Allied health professionals
CSCI	Commission for Social Care Inspection
DH	Department of Health
GP	General practice/practitioner
LAA	Local area agreement
LSP	Local strategic partnership
NHS	National Health Service
NSF	National Service Framework
OT	Occupational therapy
PBC	Practice-based commissioning
PBR	Payment by results
PCG/PCO/PCT	Primary care group/organisation/trust
PHCT	Primary health care team
SHA	Strategic health authority
SSD	Social services department

All web references in the following text were correct at the time of printing.

Preface

Open almost any newspaper and issues of partnership working (or lack of it) leap out at you. In extreme cases it is very rare, high-profile, front-page stories – about a child death, a mental health homicide, the abuse of a person with learning difficulties or an older person dying at home alone (see Box 0.1). Here, partnership working is quite literally a matter of life and death, and a failure to collaborate can have the most serious consequences for all involved. However, most newspaper stories focusing on social issues or on public services will inevitably include reference to partnership issues – either to the need for joint working or to a social problem that is so multifaceted that an interagency response is required. Whether it be gun crime, substance misuse, prostitution, social exclusion, regeneration, third world debt, teenage pregnancy or public health, the issues at stake are often so complex that no one agency working by itself could ever hope to provide a definitive solution (or even understand the problem in its entirety).

Box 0.1: Partnership working as a matter of life or death

Following the death of Victoria Climbié in 2000, a series of reforms have taken place in children's services to promote more effective partnerships. As the then Health Secretary explained, 'there were failures at every level and by every organisation which came into contact with Victoria Climbié. Victoria needed services that worked together. Instead the [inquiry] report says there was confusion and conflict. The only sure-fire way to break down the barriers between these services is to break down these barriers altogether' (BBC, 2003).

In services for people with learning difficulties, an investigation into alleged abuse in Cornwall found that 'working relationships between the [NHS] trust and Cornwall County Council had been poor for a considerable time' and that 'social services had little involvement in the care provided by the trust, to the detriment of

---

people with learning disabilities' (Healthcare Commission/CSCI, 2006, p 7).

In mental health services, a review of mental health homicides identified a lack of partnership working as a common feature of official inquiries (and the fourth most important out of 12 contributing factors), both in health and social care, as well as with the police, housing and the independent sector (McCulloch and Parker, 2004).

In older people's services, 'thousands of people die miserable deaths alone, uncared for and in poverty, figures suggest. A study by Liberal Democrat MP Paul Burstow found around 60 people a week die alone without the support of family and friends' (BBC, 2005). In the MP's report, factors contributing to such isolation and loneliness were thought to include bereavement, illness, physical impairment, fears for personal safety, declining self-esteem, depression, retirement and a reduction in social participation, poverty and a lack of preventative health and social services (Burstow, 2005). These findings have since been re-iterated in a report commissioned by the Department of Health and Comic Relief (O'Keeffe et al, 2007), which found that, despite references to 'partnership' in a number of policy documents, abuse and neglect of older people remains prevalent in the UK.

In the health and social care trade press, interagency issues are even more prevalent (see Box 0.2 for examples). For health and social care practitioners, if you are to make a positive and practical difference to service users and patients most of the issues you face will involve working with other professions and other organisations. For public service managers, partnership working is likely to occupy an increasing amount of your time and your budget, and arguably requires different skills and approaches to those prioritised in traditional single agency training and development courses. For social policy students and policy makers, many of the issues you study and/or try to resolve inevitably involve multiple professions and multiple organisations – in both health and social care, and in the public, private and voluntary sectors. Put simply, people do not live their lives according to the categories we create in our welfare services (and in subsequent professional training and organisational structures) – real-life problems are nearly always messier, more complex, harder to define and more difficult to resolve than this.

Box 0.2: Partnership working in everyday health and social care practice

At the time of writing, the latest edition of *Community Care* magazine contained news items, opinion pieces and features about:

- child poverty and well-being
- a child death and allegations of insufficient interagency communication
- poor integration of services for children and/or young people
- the experience of people with learning difficulties in the criminal justice system
- services for children whose parents have a substance misuse problem.

Nursing Times contained pieces on:

- the link between mental health and substance misuse
- the education of nurses working in nursing homes
- the physical health of people with mental health problems
- joint working between the National Health Service (NHS) and the private sector to improve access to healthcare
- new ways of working to provide surgery and diagnostics in community settings.

In addition, *The Guardian* contained stories about:

- the link between substance misuse and crime
- gun crime in inner-city areas
- policies to tackle traffic congestion in busy cities
- the potential privatisation of the probation service
- parental mental health and the impact on children.

Policy context

In response, national and local policy increasingly calls for enhanced and more effective partnership working as a potential solution. While such calls for more joint working can be inconsistent, grudgingly made and/or overly aspirational, the fact remains that collaboration between different professions and different organisations is increasingly seen as the norm (rather than as an exception to the rule). With most new funding and most new policy initiatives, there is usually a requirement that local agencies work together to bid for new resources or to deliver the required service, and various Acts of Parliament place statutory duties of partnership on a range of public bodies. As an example of the growing importance of partnership working, the word 'partnership' was recorded 6,197 times in 1999 in official parliamentary records, compared to just 38 times in 1989 (Jupp, 2000, p 7). When we repeated this exercise for the publication of this book series, we found that there were 17,912 parliamentary references to 'partnership' in 2006 alone (although this falls to 11,319 when you remove references to legislation on civil partnerships that was being debated at the time) (for further details see www.publications.parliament.uk/pa/cm/cmhansrd.htm).

In 1998, the Department of Health issued a consultation document on future relationships between health and social care. Entitled *Partnership in action*, the document proposed various ways of promoting more effective partnerships, basing these on a scathing but extremely accurate critique of single agency ways of working (DH, 1998, p 3):

> All too often when people have complex needs spanning both health and social care good quality services are sacrificed for sterile arguments about boundaries. When this happens people, often the most vulnerable in our society ... and those who care for them find themselves in the no man's land between health and social services. This is not what people want or need. It places the needs of the organisation above the needs of the people they are there to serve. It is poor

organisation, poor practice, poor use of taxpayers' money
– it is unacceptable.

Whatever you might think about subsequent policy and practice, the
fact that a government document sets out such a strongly worded
statement of its beliefs and guiding principles is extremely important.
In fact, there is often reason to question whether current commitments
to the principle of partnership working are really as benign and well
meaning as this quote implies. Like any significant change in policy
emphasis and focus, the current trend towards closer joint working
is probably the result of multiple interrelated factors (and many of
these are explored throughout this current book series). However,
the fact remains that partnership working is no longer an option (if it
ever was), but a core part of all public services and all public service
professions.

Aim and ethos of the 'Better partnership working' series

Against this background, this book (and the overall series of which it
is part) aims to provide an introduction to partnership working via a
series of accessible 'how to' books (see Box 0.3). Designed to be short
and easy to use, they are nevertheless evidence-based and theoretically
robust. A key aim is to provide *rigour and relevance* via books that:

- offer some practical support to those working with other agencies
  and professions and provide some helpful frameworks with which
  to make sense of the complexity that partnership working entails;
- summarise current policy and research in a detailed but accessible
  manner;
- provide practical but also evidence-based recommendations for
  policy and practice.

Box 0.3: The series at a glance

- *Partnership working in health and social care* (Jon Glasby and Helen Dickinson)
- *Managing and leading in inter-agency settings* (Edward Peck and Helen Dickinson)
- *Interprofessional education and training* (John Carpenter and Helen Dickinson)
- *Working in teams* (Kim Jelphs and Helen Dickinson)
- *Evaluating outcomes in health and social care* (Helen Dickinson)

While each book is cross-referenced with others in the series, each is designed to act as a standalone text with all you need to know as a student, a practitioner, a manager or a policy maker to make sense of the difficulties inherent in partnership working. In particular, the series aims to provide some practical examples to illustrate the more theoretical knowledge of social policy students, and some theoretical material to help make sense of the practical experiences and frustrations of frontline workers and managers.

Although there is a substantial and growing literature on partnership working (see, for example, Hudson, 2000; Payne, 2000; Rummery and Glendinning, 2000; Balloch and Taylor, 2001; 6 et al, 2002; Glendinning et al, 2002a; Sullivan and Skelcher, 2002; Barrett et al, 2005), most current books are either broad edited collections, very theoretical books inaccessible for students and practitioners, or texts focusing on partnership working for specific user groups. Where more practical, accessible and general texts exist, these typically lack any real depth or evidence base – in many ways little more than partnership 'cookbooks' that give you apparently simple instructions that are meant to lead to the perfect and desired outcome. In practice, anyone who has studied or worked in health and social care knows that partnership working can be both frustrating and messy – even if you follow the so-called 'rules', then the end result is often hard to predict, ambiguous and likely to provoke different reactions from different agencies and professions. In contrast, this book series seeks to offer a more 'warts and all' approach to the topic, acknowledging the practice realities that practitioners, managers and policy makers face in the real world.

Wherever possible the series focuses on key concepts, themes and frameworks rather than on the specifics of current policy and current organisational structures (which inevitably change frequently). As a result the series will hopefully be of use to readers in all four countries of the UK. That said, where structures and key policies have to be mentioned, they will typically be those in place in England. While the focus of the series is on public sector health and social care, it is important to note from the outset that current policy and practice also emphasises a range of additional partnerships and relationships, including:

- broader partnerships (for example with services such as transport and leisure in adult services and with education and youth justice in children's services);
- collaboration not just between services, but also between professionals and people who use services;
- relationships between the public, private and voluntary sectors.

As a result, many of the frameworks and concepts in each book (although summarised here in a public sector health and social care context) will also be relevant to a broader range of practitioners, students, services and service users.

Ultimately, the current emphasis on partnership working means that everything about public services – their organisation and culture, professional education and training, inspection and quality assurance – will have to change. Against this background, we hope that this series of books is a contribution, however small, to these changes.

Jon Glasby and Helen Dickinson, Series Editors
Health Services Management Centre, School of Public Policy,
University of Birmingham

1

What is partnership working and why does it matter?

In almost every walk of life, there is a balance to be struck between the expertise of the single practitioner and the need for cooperation, collaboration and coordination. This is evident in many of life's most stressful events – when you move house, for example, you want both the solicitor and the surveyor to be experts in their respective fields, but you also want all those involved to communicate and to cooperate so that the overall process goes smoothly. Equally, when you fit a new kitchen, you want a qualified gas fitter to install the boiler and an experienced electrician to handle the electrics – if the wrong person tries to do these things then the consequences could be fatal. However, you also want someone in overall control of the project so that there are no unnecessary delays and so that the person tiling the floor comes after the person who has to dig up the floor to lay some pipes. With both these examples – moving house and fitting a kitchen – there is scope for some of the key players to blur the boundary of their role and sometimes take on broader tasks, but there are also elements of the process that are only appropriate for a qualified expert.

If all this is true of everyday life, it is even more the case in health and social care, where the consequences of getting it wrong can be equally as fatal as the potential for faulty wiring or gas leaks in the examples above. When you move house or fit a kitchen, it can be incredibly frustrating when things go wrong – often you can feel completely powerless to do anything constructive and simply have to wait until problems resolve themselves. If delays leave you without temporary accommodation or without water and power for some time, you incur extra costs, significant disruption to your daily routine and a substantial impact on your quality of life. While the same is true in health and social care, the key difference is the potentially life and death nature of people's contact with formal services. When you are seriously ill and need surgical intervention, waiting or negotiating with busy professionals is often not an option – if you need treatment now, then you really need it. Even in the community, people frequently approach services only reluctantly when they have exhausted every other avenue, and are often tired, scared and in desperate need of someone to help them understand what is happening to them, to think through possible solutions and to support them to get what they need. When you are ill, in pain or facing potentially life-changing events, then being passed from pillar to post by the very services that are meant to be supporting you can be a soul-destroying and extremely negative experience.

Against this background, this chapter explores the growing literature on partnership working in order to produce a practical (albeit tentative) definition of key terms and to help readers think through the different types of relationship they may need with different types of profession and organisation in order to deliver particular outcomes for service users and patients. In the process, this discussion links to some of the frameworks set out later in the book, and includes some practical case studies of health and social care communities that have developed close working relationships, including both positive and negative examples. The chapter concludes by summarising the current policy context, highlighting the problematic nature of the health and social care divide and ways in which this boundary has shifted over time. In the process, this chapter draws out some of the negative implications of the divide for users, practitioners and organisations.

Key terms

Part of the problem with 'partnership working' is that the term itself can mean all things to all people. As Leathard (1994, p 5) has vividly observed, this area is a 'terminological quagmire' (demonstrated by the 52 separate terms that Leathard then lists to illustrate her point), a classic example of the 'definitional chaos' described by Ling (2000, p 83). In many ways this is because the issues at stake are complex (and often mean that we have to depart from traditional ways of doing things). However, this confusion is also made worse by the rhetoric in national policy documents that tend to talk about collaboration in all kinds of unspecified ways as being a 'good thing' that leads to all kinds of different and better outcomes for people who use services. While the issue of outcomes is discussed in more detail below and in the final book in the current series, *Evaluating outcomes in health and social care* by Helen Dickinson, there is little doubt that 'collaboration' and 'partnership' are current buzzwords (much like 'community' in the early 1990s or 'empowerment' and 'involvement' in the late 1990s). The classic example here is the notion of 'public–private partnerships' (PPPs), which are not partnerships at all (see below for further discussion), but which sound much more palatable and much less alien to the public sector because of the use of the word 'partnership' in the title.

In many ways, however, the examples of *community*, *empowerment* and *involvement* above offer some useful insights. While these terms are over-used, used imprecisely and often misused, they all refer to some sort of underlying concept or principle that seems important and worth striving for. We may not know exactly what the term 'empowerment' means, but we still think it is important and we often know it when we see it. Similarly, the term 'partnership working' refers to something highly significant and something worth trying to define and understand. Thus, even those commentators who have criticised the lack of precision in current policy still end up having to use some kind of similar term. A good example here is the King's Fund's helpful discussion paper, *Partnerships under pressure*, which quite rightly identifies a number of problems with the term 'partnership' (Banks, 2002, p 5):

> The term "partnerships" is increasingly losing credibility, as it has become a catch-all for a wide range of concepts and a panacea for a multitude of ills. Partnerships can cover a wide spectrum of relationships and can operate at different levels, from informally taking account of other players, to having

a constructive dialogue, working together on a project or service, joint commissioning and strategic alliances.

Despite this, the remainder of the discussion paper provides further definitional clarity, but continues to use the term 'partnership' throughout the rest of the document. In short, terms such as 'partnership working' may not always be very helpful, but they are often the best terms we have, and if they did not exist we would probably have to invent them.

Part of the difficulty in being more precise about key terms is that most writers criticise current approaches, then produce their own definition. While this is understandable, it means that there are a large number of definitions available, and that few commentators mean exactly the same thing by the same terms. For students and for frontline workers this seems unhelpful at best, and runs the risk of complicating further an already complex issue. Rather than repeat the same mistake, this book sets out some examples of basic definitions that we have found helpful (see Box 1.1), and tries to summarise some of the key features that we (and most writers) have in mind when talking about these issues. More important than the actual definition employed, however, is the way in which we distinguish 'partnerships' from other ways of organising public services (and we discuss this in more detail below). For people using this book to study or in practice, the key issue is to check out that, whatever definition is being used, all key partners mean and understand the same thing (and this is a central feature of subsequent discussion).

Box 1.1: Helpful definitions

In a key introductory textbook, Sullivan and Skelcher (2002) suggest that key features of partnerships are that they:

- involve negotiation between people from different agencies committed to working together over more than the short term;

- aim to secure the delivery of benefits or added value that could not have been provided by any single agency acting alone or through the employment of others (that is, shared goals);
- include a formal articulation of a purpose and a plan to bind partners together.

For Glendinning et al (2002a, p 3), a minimal definition of partnership working requires the involvement of 'at least two agents or agencies with at least some sort of common interests or interdependencies; and would probably also require a relationship between them that involves a degree of trust, equality or reciprocity'.

In contrast, for the Audit Commission (2002) the focus is more on 'whole systems working', whereby:

- services are organised around the needs of the service user;
- services recognise that they are interdependent and that action in one part of the system will have a 'knock-on effect' somewhere else;
- agencies develop shared vision, objectives, action, resources and risks;
- users experience services as seamless.

For Alex Scott-Samuel, partnership working is often better described as 'putting mutual loathing aside in order to get your hands on the money' (quoted in Powell and Dowling, 2006, p 308).

For Powell and Dowling (2006, p 305), partnership working involves 'the indefinable in pursuit of the unachievable'.

For Thomson and Perry (1998, p 409), 'collaboration is like cottage cheese. It occasionally smells bad and separates easily'.

While we use phrases such as *partnership working*, *interagency collaboration* and *joint working* interchangeably, these various definitions highlight a number of key issues and principles that are worth stressing (and that readers should bear in mind as they read the rest of this book):

- Behind most definitions is a sense of *added value* – an ability to achieve something together that could not be achieved separately (perhaps encapsulated in the notion of 'the whole being greater than the sum of its parts').

- Also significant is a sense of *reciprocity* (that is, for the relationship to be mutually beneficial, and for some sort of sharing of potential risks or drawbacks).

- Several definitions emphasise some sort of *formal and ongoing relationship* – for some in Box 1.1, collaboration and partnership are clearly a journey and, while they may not yet know where this will lead, the agencies involved must recognise that this is a route they need to travel together.

- In many ways, an acid test is the subsequent experience of *people who use services* – perhaps something is only an effective partnership if it feels like it to people on the receiving end.

- Implicit in several definitions is the notion of partnership and collaboration as *voluntary* in nature – based on trust, equality and recognition of interdependence rather than on compulsion. While we return to the issue of so-called 'forced partnerships' later in the book, a central component of collaboration for us is that individual partners *retain the right of exit* (that is, if the collaboration is not perceived to be delivering desired outcomes for both partners, then they have the right to leave that collaboration). This is clearly very different to other ways of working – in a market-based relationship, for example, there will be a formal contract binding agencies together and often preventing exit, except in very tightly defined circumstances.

- While most literature on collaboration is positive, some definitions (albeit tongue in cheek) hint at *possible negatives* and *cynical motivations* that should warn us against always seeing partnership as a 'good thing' (see below for further discussion).

Markets, hierarchies and networks: a brief overview

Although it can be difficult to be clear exactly what different commentators mean by terms such as 'collaboration' and 'partnership', it can often help to try to distinguish between these concepts and other ways of delivering public services. Typically, services tend to be organised on the basis of *hierarchies*, *markets* or *networks* (see Box 1.2), and part of the problem is that the term 'partnership' can be used to describe all three. In the UK, many current welfare services began life in the voluntary and community sector, with various 19th-century philanthropists and charities gradually developing new ways of responding to the social problems created by rapid industrialisation and urbanisation. While the development of state welfare is described in more detail elsewhere (see, for example, Hill, 2000; Fraser, 2003), it was often the voluntary sector that pioneered developments such as old-age pensions, child health services, adult education, affordable housing and practical support for older and disabled people, many of which became part of a state-led and publicly funded welfare system following the reforms of the 1940s. In many ways, this was an era of *hierarchy*, with large government departments responsible for a series of (often quite separate) welfare services, each with their own regional and local delivery structures. Authority in such a system was very top-down, with staff at ground level reporting up to a lead officer, who themselves would report upwards.

From the late 1970s, a series of national and international economic crises prompted a radical rethink, and the Conservative governments of Margaret Thatcher (1979-90) began a process of *market-based reform*. According to this ideology, a very large public sector had become massively inefficient, consuming too much of the nation's resources and serving the interests of staff and welfare professionals rather than people receiving services. In response, public services were reformed according to market principles, with the public sector increasingly focused on purchasing services from a growing range of public, private and voluntary organisations, rather than providing them all itself 'in-

–

7

house'. Thus, in the National Health Service (NHS), a 'purchaser–provider split' meant that health authorities were increasingly to pay for the hospital services provided to local people by a series of new and more self-financing NHS hospital trusts. In social care, moreover, the community care reforms of the early 1990s increasingly saw social workers as assessors and care managers, identifying and meeting needs from a menu of services (that could be provided by a range of different organisations and not just by in-house social care services). In a market-based system like this, the emphasis was very much on assessing needs (both of the population and of the individual) and securing the services to meet those needs from the best available supplier. While 'best' here could include considerations of cost, quality and responsiveness to service user needs, there was arguably a tendency to focus on cost as the main criterion. Under a market, moreover, service providers have a strong incentive to change their behaviour in order to be efficient and competitive, but there is also a risk of increased costs and complexity when trying to establish and manage the market, to judge quality and to ensure standards. Where services are very specialist, there can often be a risk of a single provider monopolising all provision (which then prevents competition and can remove incentives to remain cost-effective and efficient). More generally, those services better able to adapt to the market also tend to out-survive competitors who struggle to change – while this can remove some poor quality services, it can also lead to a situation where larger and larger companies take over the majority of suppliers and where small organisations can no longer afford to keep up.

More recently, interest has grown in the concepts of partnerships and of *networks*. In many ways, this was a response to the practical implications of the changes of the 1980s and the 1990s. As a result of previous market reforms, public services became increasingly fragmented, with a growing split between commissioners of services and providers from the public, private and voluntary sectors. This is described by Sullivan and Skelcher (2002, pp 15-20) in terms of 'the hollowed-out state', with the government continuing to be responsible for identifying what services are needed and much less involved in

–

delivering this itself. At the very time when policy was starting to focus on more complex, cross-cutting social problems, therefore, mechanisms for responding to such need were increasingly diverse and fragmented. Against this background, the solution, perhaps unsurprisingly, was the notion of 'joined-up solutions to joined-up problems', with a much greater emphasis on interagency working and partnership as a means of coordinating something of a patchwork quilt of services. Within this context, the term *network* is often used to describe a way of organising based much more on informal relationships, trust and reciprocity (see Box 1.2).

Box 1.2: Hierarchies, markets and networks

A *hierarchy* is often a single organisation (perhaps a large bureaucracy), with top-down rules, procedures and statutes that govern how the organisation works.

In contrast, a *market* involves multiple organisations exchanging goods and services based on competition and price.

A *network* is often seen as lying in between these two approaches, with multiple organisations coming together more informally, often based on interpersonal relationships or a shared outlook (Thompson et al, 1991; 6 et al, 2006).

As helpful shorthand, Rodríguez et al (2007, p 158) have caricatured these approaches as being about:

- rules (hierarchy)
- incentives (market)
- interactions (network)

Markets, hierarchies and networks: the more complex reality

Of course, the problem with the brief overview above is that it runs the risk of over-simplifying a more complex reality. While the distinction between 1940s-1970s hierarchy, 1980s markets and post-1997 networks is a useful shorthand, it portrays the evolution of services in a very linear way. In practice, we believe that the shift from hierarchies to markets to networks may be more cyclical. Thus, over time traditional hierarchies run the risk of being seen to be very bureaucratic, very large, very expensive and very unresponsive to need. While there is no inherent reason why a hierarchy should be like this, the temptation in our political system has been to break up these hierarchies and turn them into markets, thus using choice, competition and 'customer power' to make services change. Over time, markets can be seen as creating too much fragmentation, and networks become a more attractive concept – bringing together different agencies and stakeholders to work in new more cross-cutting ways. However, as the issue at stake rises up the political agenda, it can reach a stage where it is deemed to be so important that we no longer trust networks to handle it, and we quickly turn it back into a hierarchy (which we feel we can manage and control more directly). From here the cycle begins again. While this sounds very abstract, some more concrete examples in Box 1.3 show how this can happen in practice.

While this has been quite a detailed and complex summary, the debate is an important one because of our tendency to use words such as 'partnership' very imprecisely to refer to hierarchies, markets and networks all at the same time (see Box 1.4). Thus, many current health and social care 'partnerships' are actually hierarchies – they may bring together health and social care, but they do so in large, public sector bureaucracies with a chief executive and a board, a senior management team and all the systems and processes of a standard hierarchical organisation. Equally, some market-based relationships – for example, PPPs – are (wrongly) described as 'partnerships', perhaps because they can involve long-term relationships but also because it sounds more attractive and politically acceptable. Similarly, many networks share many features with the key definitions in Box 1.1 above, and represent a particular form of partnership.

Box 1.3: Cyclical changes in the way we organise services

Arguably, health, and to a lesser extent, social care, have a cultural preference for hierarchy, yet a growing distrust of bureaucracy and over-centralisation. Over time, a number of initiatives have arisen as networks yet have quickly become so important that we have turned them back into hierarchies. At the same time, some hierarchies have seemed so large and potentially inefficient that we have broken them up via market mechanisms. Examples include:

- *Changes in mental health services*, where initial community mental health teams (which were very loose, informal and bottom-up collaborations) have become increasingly hierarchical as mental health has become more of a political priority. Under current policy, there is now detailed guidance as to what kind of teams we need, staff numbers and caseloads, in a much more hierarchical, managed system.

- In *child protection*, a similar shift from network-based area child protection arrangements to much more hierarchical safeguarding children boards took place following a number of high profile child deaths and a landmark inquiry by Lord Laming into the death of Victoria Climbié (Laming, 2003).

- *Health Action Zones* (HAZs) often began as networks to bring people together to develop innovative responses to cross-cutting problems such as health inequalities and poor health. Over time, these initiatives were given more and more central targets, were subjected to tighter central control and began to appoint their own 'directors'. As they began to be perceived as 'not delivering' or as too large and inefficient, many HAZs began to contact out their work to the market.

Box 1.4: 'Partnership working': meaning all things to all people

Some health and social care partnerships are actually hierarchies – a care trust or a mental health partnership trust, for example. While we discuss the example of the integrated mental health trust created in Somerset in Chapter 2 later, this was initially seen as a ground-breaking example of collaboration and partnership. With hindsight, it was actually a network in the process of turning into a hierarchy (albeit an integrated one), and the language used to describe this important innovation should perhaps have been more precise (with the benefit of hindsight).

Partnerships UK is a PPP formed by HM Treasury in 2000 to invest in public services and infrastructure. With a majority stake (51%) held by the private sector and the remainder retained by the government, it raises capital from shareholders such as banks, building societies and other private sector companies. As such, it might more accurately be described as a market-based relationship.

In the NHS, several medical specialities have developed clinical networks, with professionals in areas such as cancer, heart disease and diabetes coming together as a network to develop more patient-focused care across primary and secondary healthcare services.

The upshot of all this is twofold:

• When practitioners, local organisations and policy makers talk about collaboration and partnership, they often mean very different things by the same terms. As a result, it is crucial to be abundantly clear about the kind of relationship you are talking about.
• Ultimately, what matters most is what you are trying to achieve for service users and for your organisation. Only when you are clear about what you want to achieve can you move on to consider who

you need to work with and what kind of relationships you may need. This is discussed in further detail in Chapter 4, with various frameworks to help clarify these issues and to guide decision making.

Why does partnership working matter?

Just as there are a wide range of definitions of 'partnership', so too there are a myriad of checklists that set out the supposed advantages of partnership working (see Box 1.5 for some prominent examples). Unfortunately, such lists tend to be unremittingly positive, emphasising perceived benefits without citing any evidence for the claims made and without listing any of the potential negatives. The extent to which current evidence is able to identify whether partnerships are effective (and if so, for whom and under which circumstances) is explored later in Chapters 2 and 3 (as well as in another book in this series, *Evaluating outcomes in health and social care*, by Helen Dickinson). While partnership working seems like a better way of doing things than in single agencies, it is actually quite hard to understand whether this is true and, if so, why and how. Certainly, many of the claims made in Box 1.5 (although they may well be true) are not based on clear-cut and unambiguous evidence, and approaching a topic such as partnership working with a healthy scepticism may be a good way forward. Even more important than this, however, is the need to place the current emphasis on partnership working in a broader context in order to understand where it has come from and why it has developed the way it has.

Often, when the world changes, we like to think it is because of the power of ideas – because somebody somewhere has had a vision of how things could be different and has convinced enough people to make this start to happen. Unfortunately, all the available evidence suggests that the power of ideas can be limited by what it seems possible to think. In other words, people are predisposed to 'have' and accept new ideas by the context in which they live and work, by the unwritten rules about why life, the universe and everything is the way it is.

Box 1.5: Why work in partnership?

For the Audit Commission (1998, p 9):

> ... there are five main reasons why agencies develop partnerships:
>
> - To deliver co-ordinated packages of services to individuals
> - To tackle so-called 'wicked issues' [that is, cross-cutting, complex problems where we do not really know the best way of responding to the issue at stake]
> - To reduce the impact of organisational fragmentation and minimise the impact of any perverse incentives that arise from it
> - To bid for, or gain access to, new resources, and
> - To meet a statutory requirement.

For Payne (2000, p 41), there are six purposes for multiprofessional work: bringing together skills; sharing information; achieving continuity of care; apportioning and ensuring responsibility and accountability; coordination in planning resources; and coordination in delivering resources for professionals to apply for the benefit of service users.

For the Department of Health (1998, p 5):

> Those most likely to suffer from the failure of the current system are the most vulnerable – frail older people, adults or children with mental health problems, learning or physical disabilities. They require support from both health and social services because of the changing and ongoing nature of their needs. Our proposals, promised in the NHS White Paper, are designed to help those most in need by ensuring better delivery of the services they want when they want them.

Thus, at any given time, some ideas and changes seem feasible and/or desirable, but this is governed by the current economic, political, social and cultural context in which we are located.

In terms of partnership working, the dramatic rise in the importance of this topic can seem at first glance like a vindication for the power of ideas. If we revisit the 1998 *Partnership in action* quote from the preface, one interpretation is of a government that has diagnosed a key problem in current services and that is taking a decisive and principled stand to put things right (DH, 1998, p 3):

> All too often when people have complex needs spanning both health and social care good quality services are sacrificed for sterile arguments about boundaries. When this happens people, often the most vulnerable in our society ... and those who care for them find themselves in the no man's land between health and social services. This is not what people want or need. It places the needs of the organisation above the needs of the people they are there to serve. It is poor organisation, poor practice, poor use of taxpayers' money – it is unacceptable.

While this is a powerful rationale, an additional explanation is that the context is currently right for partnership working to be seen as a 'good thing' and as the best way forward for health and social care services. This is a complex issue beyond the scope of the current book series (although for a more detailed account of these changes in an international context see Dickinson and Glasby, 2008). For present purposes, Box 1.6 sets out some of the key factors that we feel have contributed to the current emphasis on partnership working, although this list is neither definitive nor uncontested.

Box 1.6: Factors promoting a focus on partnership working

When a new way of working becomes a core feature of policy (in the UK and in many other developed countries), it is often the result of a series of wider and interrelated political, economic and social factors. For example, the current emphasis on partnership working could be variously attributed to some combination of the following factors:

- the increased fragmentation of services following the implementation of various market-based approaches to public services;
- the emphasis placed on 'customer satisfaction' by current political philosophies;
- the growth of various civil rights movements (around 'race', gender and disability), with service user-led organisations increasingly calling for services that enable them to lead chosen lifestyles (and for services that fit their lives, not the other way round);
- demographic changes (with older, more diverse and more mobile populations) and advances in medicine and technology, leading to a need to deliver services in new and more cost-effective ways;
- rising public expectations and a growing challenge to traditional professional power.

Again, this is much more than an academic exercise – such issues matter because they help to explain why partnership working is being promoted, why frontline practitioners experience some of the frustrations they do, why different policies can often seem contradictory in nature and why it is so difficult to evaluate partnership working. Put simply, if people working in partnerships have very different (and often subconscious) motivations for doing so, then we should not be surprised if the results are ambiguous, unclear and contested.

Policy context

In many ways, both current and previous attempts to promote more effective partnerships arise directly out of the underlying assumptions that underpin our current welfare system (for an overview, see Means and Smith, 1998; Means et al, 2003; Glasby and Littlechild, 2004). Under the 1940s legislation that set up the current welfare state, it was assumed that it was possible to distinguish between people who were *sick* (that is, people we see as having *health needs* that are met by the NHS free at the point of delivery) and people who were merely *frail or disabled* (who we see as having *social care needs* that fall under the remit of local authority adult social services and that are frequently subject to a means test and to user charges). This underlying distinction then results in two separate agencies with very different structures, priorities, financial systems and ways of working, and all the subsequent complexities that partnership working entails (see Box 1.7 for a summary of key differences between health and social care). Over time, there have been many attempts to overcome this boundary – from joint consultative committees in the 1970s to hospital discharge protocols in the 1990s, and from local agreements over the boundary between home care and district nursing to a raft of national guidance on the difference between long-term care, free personal care and NHS continuing healthcare (for a more detailed discussion, see Glasby and Littlechild, 2004). However, the fact remains that this divide continues to exist and continues to cause problems for policy makers, practitioners and service users alike. While recent policy has become much more sophisticated at hiding and blurring the health and social care divide, its influence is no less profound than it ever was.

> **Box 1.7: The health and social care divide**
>
> * Healthcare is accountable nationally to the Secretary of State for Health; social care is part of local government and accountable to locally elected councillors.

—

17

- Healthcare is free at the point of delivery; (adult) social care often entails a means test and user charges.
- Healthcare tends to be based on general practitioner (GP) registration (which is often based on catchment areas around individual practices); social care is based on strict local authority geographical boundaries.
- Healthcare is often dominated by medicine and looks to the sciences for its education and training; social care is much more influenced by the social sciences.
- Healthcare often focuses on curing the individual; social care places greater emphasis on seeing the individual in context and potentially intervening socially and politically rather than always individually.

In children's services, the nature of the debate is slightly different. While the health and social care divide continues to be a source of potential fragmentation, a more prominent fault line is between the education system (with its emphasis on attainment and qualifications) and social care (with its emphasis on protection and well-being). As with adult health and social care, such approaches are arguably two sides of the same coin, and intuitively it would seem as if feeling safe and happy should be a fundamental building block for subsequent educational attainment. However, this is not the way our system is structured, and both education and children's social care have historically been governed by different government departments, different organisational structures, different financial systems and different cultures and values. Nowhere is this more apparent than in recent performance measures – with schools assessed on the educational achievements of their pupils, there is an incentive built in to the system to work with those pupils most likely to score well in their examinations. While education may therefore be trying to raise the number of children passing their GCSEs with grades A–C, social care is working to protect and include many children and young people who could be seen as 'dragging results down' in a system geared to performance alone. Although this is a massive over-simplification of a much more complicated reality, it is a recognisable over-simplification and may contain more than a degree of truth behind the parody.

However, we should be careful about seeing the emphasis on partnership working as the sole product of the problematic health/ social care or education/children's social care divide. No matter how their services are structured or funded, most, if not all, developed countries are struggling with the same issues (see, for example, Johri et al, 2003; Leichsenring and Alaszewski, 2004; Kodner, 2006; Dickinson and Glasby, 2008), and even the briefest of trawls across the experience of other systems suggests that there is no such thing as the perfect organisational structure (see below for further discussion). No matter where we put the boundary, organisational divisions will always exist, and it depends on your perspective as to whether current boundaries are more or less helpful. As Leutz (1999) has argued in an often-cited commentary on partnership working, 'your integration is my fragmentation'. Wherever the boundary is located, the trick is in how best to manage it and limit any negative implications for people who use services (and it is this that lies behind the current book and the wider book series).

Arising out of this policy context, health and social care in the early 21st century are developing and drawing on a range of different forms of collaboration as they seek to meet the demands being made of them. Although Box 1.8 provides some of the more prominent examples, we should again guard against the danger of seeing partnership and collaboration as inherently 'a good thing'. While each health and social care community is trying to find the best and most locally appropriate way forward through the complexities they face, there are many negative as well as positive examples (see Box 1.9), and the evidence base behind current collaborations is thin to say the least. Against this background, the remainder of this book (and the wider series of which it is part) seeks to summarise the key messages from research and to provide a series of broader theoretical frameworks so that busy students, practitioners, managers and policy makers can make as much sense as possible of these difficult issues and hopefully be better equipped as they work with partner agencies. However, underlying the remainder of the book and the series as a whole is the issue of *outcomes* – being clear about what health and social care partners are trying to achieve for their own organisations and for people who use services, about which options are available to them, and about which partnerships and with whom may work best in any given situation. Ultimately, this can be paraphrased as a key question that remains largely unanswered in the current policy context, and that all potential 'partners' would do well to ask themselves – if partnership is the answer, what is the question?

Box 1.8: Examples of current partnerships

Under the 1999 Health Act, health and social care can use one or more of three new 'flexibilities' (the ability to pool their funding, create an integrated service provider and/or to nominate one partner as a lead commissioner) (for the results of a national evaluation see Glendinning et al, 2002b).

Under the 2001 Health and Social Care Act, health and social care communities can create a care trust – a single integrated organisation. These are essentially NHS bodies with social care responsibilities delegated to them, and can either focus on providing services (for example, building on a previous NHS mental health trust) or on providing and commissioning (for example, building on a previous NHS primary care trust [PCT]). Unpopular with local government, there remain few care trusts and their future is uncertain (for an introductory textbook see Glasby and Peck, 2003).

In children's services, a children's trust brings together all services for children and young people, underpinned by a duty to cooperate set out in the 2004 Children Act. In addition, key policies for joining up children's services include a common assessment framework, work to develop the role of a lead professional and greater information sharing (for results of a national evaluation of children's trusts see University of East Anglia, 2007).

Short of such structural solutions, other collaborations take the form of joint appointments between health and social care, integrated management structures, single assessment processes and 'one-stop shop' entry points into the health and social care system.

Away from health and social care, local strategic partnerships (LSPs) bring together the full range of partners from the public, private, voluntary and community sectors to provide an overarching framework for improving the social, economic and environmental well-being of an area. More recently, local area agreements (LAAs) are a means by which local areas can coordinate their activities, negotiate local outcomes that they wish to prioritise and simplify central funding streams (for the results of relevant national evaluations see studies funded by the former ODPM, 2005a, 2007; ODPM and Department of Transport, 2006).

For further information on these models, visit:

- www.dh.gov.uk
- www.dfes.gov.uk
- www.communities.gov.uk
- www.integratedcarenetwork.gov.uk

Box 1.9: The negatives of partnership working

In Wiltshire, high-profile financial difficulties and an apparent breakdown in communication between health and social care led to the dismantling of long-standing partnership arrangements and high-profile media discussion (see, for example, O'Hara, 2006).

In Cornwall, inspectors found evidence of abuse and poor practice in a number of learning disability services. Although these were provided by a 'partnership trust', the inspectors concluded that 'working relations between the trust and Cornwall County

Council have been poor for a considerable time' (Healthcare Commission/CSCI, 2006, p 7).

Tackling delayed transfers of care has become a key government priority, yet the 'partnership' arrangements put in place to respond to this issue arguably focus unfairly on one partner, giving hospitals the ability to 'fine' their social care partners for inappropriate delays (see CSCI, 2004, 2005; see also Chapter 3 for further discussion).

In Manchester, an abuse scandal in a newly formed care trust prompted significant criticism from national inspectors, who questioned the readiness of previous organisations to form a care trust, expressed concerns over relations between the care trust and other partners, and argued that the process of forming a care trust may have detracted senior management time away from service issues and quality of care (CHI, 2003).

In Barking and Dagenham, the local authority and PCT had initially appointed a single chief executive of the PCT/executive director of health and social care, yet this broke down after a negative star rating of the PCT amid significant negative media coverage (see, for example, Batty, 2003).

Interestingly, some of these examples of negative aspects of partnership working relate to issues of *process* (how well agencies work together), while others refer to negative *outcomes* for service users. This is a key distinction that recurs throughout this book and that is explored in more detail below.

Reflective exercises

1. Think of a situation in your private life where you have received services that you felt should have been working together on your behalf more effectively (for example, when you moved house, when you had a car accident and had to liaise with multiple insurance companies, when you experienced a break-in and had to link with the police, your insurance and a loss adjustor). How coordinated was this process? What helped and what hindered? How did it feel to be on the receiving end of such services? What avenues and mechanisms existed to help you get what you needed? How positive or negative an experience was this, and why?

2. What does the term 'partnership working' mean to you? Share this with a friend or a colleague from a different background to compare and contrast your different definitions.

3. What 'partnerships' exist in your local area, and to what extent are they based on hierarchies, markets or networks?

4. Think of a child or an adult that you have worked with or read about. How easy it is it to divide their needs up into health, social care or educational needs, and how meaningful would this be from the point of view of the person concerned?

5. In a situation where you have worked with somebody from a different organisational or professional background, what outcome did it achieve for your organisation, for you and for people who use services? What costs or negatives were there, and was the outcome you achieved together worth it?

Note: All the reflective exercises in this book assume that practitioners will be able to draw on first-hand experiences from their work. For students who may not yet have experienced such issues, these exercises work just as well if you apply them to any other interagency or collaborative situation – for example, playing in a sports team, organising a student society or coming together to do group work on your course.

Further reading and resources

For official health and social care policy, relevant websites include:

- Department of Health: www.dh.gov.uk
- Department for Children, Schools and Families: www.dfes.gov.uk
- Department for Communities and Local Government: www.communities.gov.uk

In addition, the government's Care Services Improvement Partnership (CSIP) (www.csip.org.uk) offers a range of practical toolkits, guidance and advice about various health and social care services, while CSIP's Integrated Care Network (www.integratedcarenetwork.gov.uk) is an essential source of information and good practice about interagency collaboration.

For guidance on good practice and on 'what works' in health and social care, see also the National Institute for Health and Clinical Excellence (NICE) (www.nice.org.uk) and the Social Care Institute for Excellence (www.scie.org.uk).

In terms of the health and social care professions, relevant professional bodies include:

- Association of Directors of Adult Social Services: www.adss.org.uk
- Association of Directors of Children's Services: www.adcs.org.uk
- British Association/College of Occupational Therapists: www.cot.org.uk
- British Association of Social Workers: www.basw.co.uk
- British Medical Association: www.bma.org.uk
- The Chartered Society of Physiotherapy: www.csp.org.uk
- NHS Alliance: www.nhsalliance.org
- The NHS Confederation: www.nhsconfed.org
- Royal College of General Practitioners: www.rcgp.org.uk
- Royal College of Nursing: www.rcn.org.uk

Key introductory textbooks on health and social care partnerships include:

- Balloch and Taylor's (2001) *Partnership working*
- Barrett et al's (2005) *Interprofessional working in health and social care*
- Glasby's (2007) *Understanding health and social care*
- Glendinning et al's (2002a) *Partnerships, New Labour and the governance of welfare*
- Sullivan and Skelcher's (2002) *Working across boundaries*

2

What does research tell us?

While partnership working is increasingly seen as a 'good thing', the evidence base underpinning such assumptions is remarkably thin. Given current commitments to evidence-based policy and practice, this rather faith-based approach to partnership working seems ironic to say the least, and we still know very little about the extent to which partnerships can deliver outcomes that other approaches cannot. In particular, much of the early partnership literature has tended to focus on how well agencies and professions are working together (or not), exploring the extent to which partners feel that they have a good relationship, trust each other and communicate regularly. While these are important issues, they concentrate very much on issues of *process* (how are we working together?), not on issues of *outcome* (does this make any difference to people using services?). As a result, despite a growing literature, our knowledge about what works for whom and in which circumstances remains extremely patchy (for more detailed discussion see *Evaluating outcomes in health and social care* by Helen Dickinson, in this series).

Against this background, this chapter reviews the claims made for partnership working, and questions the extent to which they are evidence-based. In the course of this discussion, the chapter summarises the literature on what helps and hinders partnership working, and cites practical examples from various health and social care communities. In the process, the chapter also draws on evidence from private sector mergers and acquisitions, questioning the extent to which structural change alone is able to deliver different outcomes and raising important questions about recent policy.

Neglect of outcomes in the partnership literature

As set out in Chapter 1, much of the literature on health and social care partnerships is extremely positive about the potential outcomes of partnership working for service users. Despite this, the fact remains that we know very little about the impact of partnership working, and many of the claims made above seem more faith than evidence-based. As Box 2.1 suggests, most attempts to review the literature on the outcomes of partnership conclude that too few studies focus on issues of impact and effectiveness, and that our evidence base is surprisingly under-developed. For Powell and Dowling (2006, p 305), for example, partnerships are 'the indefinable in pursuit of the unachievable', while 'there is no shortage of advice on how to "do" partnerships ... with lists of drivers, building blocks, and components..., the validity and reliability of this input into "evidence-based" policy making is less clear'.

> **Box 2.1: Neglect of outcomes in the partnership literature**
>
> A systematic review of the factors promoting and obstacles hindering joint working between health and social care concluded that:
>
> > Disappointingly, the vast majority of the studies in the review focused their attention on the process of joint working and the perceptions of those involved as to its success. Very few of the studies looked at either the prior question of why joint work should be seen as a "good thing" and therefore why it should be done, or at the subsequent question of what difference joint working made. This makes the literature somewhat circular, and almost silent on the question of effectiveness. The circularity of the literature led

> us to the disappointing conclusion that our knowledge ... has hardly moved on since the studies carried out in the late 1970s and early 1980s. (Cameron and Lart, 2003, p 15)
>
> In 2004, a review by Dowling et al (p 315) concluded that:
>
> The present authors' search of the literature has revealed the rudimentary state of the art of conceptualising, measuring and demonstrating the success of partnerships.... [Of studies included], only a few investigated whether specific partnerships had produced successful outcomes and the results were ambiguous even in these.... Thus ... knowledge of whether partnerships "work" – in the sense of producing benefits to those who pay for, provide or use services – remains very limited.

Lessons from Somerset

Indeed, such is the paucity of the evidence base that even a pioneering study of the Somerset Partnership NHS and Social Care Trust – the first such organisation of its kind in England and a national example of good practice – fails to address the issue of outcomes in full (see Peck et al, 2002). Following a 1996 review of mental health services, Somerset Health Authority and Somerset County Council took the then unique step of establishing a joint commissioning board and an integrated health and social care provider organisation. Equally unusually, Somerset took the brave step of commissioning a two-and-a-half-year evaluation of these innovations, choosing to make the lessons learned available nationally and publicly. In many ways, Somerset's vision then set the future trend for national policy and for other services, and the changes were subsequently taken up in mental health services and beyond across the country. However, from the beginning, the results of the Somerset study were ambiguous, and different interpretations exist as to the extent to which the integration was a success, and the insights into partnership working that this example provides (see Box 2.2).

Box 2.2: Different interpretations of the 'success' of partnership working

In 2000, the government's 10-year blueprint for health services, *The NHS Plan* (DH, 2000, p 71) quoted the Somerset Partnership NHS and Social Care Trust as an example of good practice, citing benefits for service users such as the existence of a single care plan, a single key worker and a unified multidisciplinary team.

In the subsequent independent evaluation published two years later, the researchers identified evidence of an initial reduction in job satisfaction, morale and role clarity, little change in levels of user satisfaction, and ambiguous results for service users (with some improvements in coordination but also concerns about the potential closure of buildings and a loss of therapeutic/support groups) (Peck et al, 2002). Although sympathetic to what was being undertaken in Somerset and respectful of the extent to which such major change could take place with relatively little upheaval, the research presented a very different picture to that of the 2000 *NHS Plan* (DH, 2000).

While the changes in Somerset were impressive in their scope and seemed to bring about some positive changes for service users, the findings of the evaluation were more nuanced. While service user satisfaction remained relatively high and consistent throughout the study, staff morale declined significantly in the short term, with concerns about workload, about a perceived loss of influence for numerically small professions and about the nature and identity of the new organisation. Although there was some evidence that service users felt that they had fewer problems keeping themselves occupied by the end of the study, it is hard to know if this was the result of the integration per se, and the problem of trying to unpick what might have happened anyway without the creation of the new trust remains. At the same time, service user concerns about the quality of acute in-patient care, about a lack of alternatives to hospital and about a lack of respect from some staff members remained similar over time (for a summary of key findings see Box 2.3).

Box 2.3: Sample findings from the Somerset Partnership NHS and Social Care Trust

- In the short term, staff found that job satisfaction, morale and role clarity reduced, although this had levelled off and in some cases reversed by the end of the study.
- While the mental health status of service users improved during this period, it is not clear whether this was attributable to the integration itself.
- While coordination improved, some users were concerned about a loss of therapeutic/support groups due to changes in the use of buildings.
- There were continued concerns about lack of alternatives to hospital in a crisis, the extent to which users were involved in negotiating care plans and the attitudes of some staff.
- While there were some improvements for carers, problems continued to exist with identifying, involving and providing information to carers.

Source: Peck et al (2002)

Against this background, debate continues about exactly what these findings mean in practice. With both positives and negatives (as well as the problem of attribution), the study raised important questions about the extent to which structural change is the best way of achieving more effective partnership (see also below for further discussion):

> The establishment of the combined Trust did not – at the conclusion of the evaluation period – appear to have delivered significant benefits that have not been delivered elsewhere in England without the transfer of social care staff to NHS employment. There is no way of knowing whether comparable changes would have been achieved in Somerset

> without the creation of the combined Trust.... Further, this
> is not to say that other, and perhaps more profound, changes
> will not follow, especially as Somerset has already put in
> place the transfer of employment of most social care staff
> that other localities may have to undertake in time. (Peck
> et al, 2002, p 41)

Equally, the concerns of service users about staff attitudes and about acute care do not appear to have been resolved by the creation of the Partnership Trust. Disappointing though this may be, in one sense it should hardly be surprising. If tackling these concerns was really the main priority of partner organisations, then arguably a different approach would have been more appropriate. Indeed, it is even possible that the integration of health and social care focused management attention so much on the *process* of partnership working that there was less emphasis on user priorities, at least in the short term.

However, perhaps the main complexity of the Somerset study, is trying to understand the overall messages that it tells us about health and social care partnerships:

- According to one reading of the Somerset story, the integration of health and social care achieved nothing that could not have been achieved with a lesser form of partnership working and less upheaval – despite all the changes, nothing essentially seemed to change for service users. If this is the case, the argument goes, it must surely raise major concerns about whether such integration is really worth the effort.

- On the other hand, other commentators look at Somerset and say that local leaders were able to pioneer new ways of working across agency boundaries and to create a new, integrated organisation – all without making anything worse for service users in the meantime. This may then have laid foundations for the future delivery of better outcomes (and we will probably now never know as a result of more recent changes in the area and in mental health services more generally, which mean that is hard to know what, if any, changes to attribute to the integration per se).

Thus, depending on your time frame and depending on your perspective, Somerset was either a major success or a major storm in a tea cup, and the extent to which partnership working really might achieve better outcomes for people who use services remains just as much a matter of faith. What is apparent, however, is that structural change can lead to potentially unintended negative outcomes in the short term, and this makes it even more important that health and social care services are clear about what they are trying to achieve and why the inevitable upheaval of organisational change is worth it in the longer run. As the lead evaluator of Somerset often says, "success often looks like failure part way through. The problem with this is that so does failure" (personal communication). As Chapter 4 discusses, this makes the need to be clear about desired outcomes (and about the best structures and processes to achieve these ends) even more fundamental. What this example and others like it also demonstrate are the difficulties inherent in evaluating partnerships and judging whether they have been 'successful' (see also *Evaluating outcomes in health and social care* by Helen Dickinson, in this series). With a range of different stakeholder perspectives and potential unintended consequences, partnerships pose a massive evaluation challenge. What this also means is that we must be careful when generalising about the outcomes of partnership working: what outcomes are we talking about, for whom, when and in what contexts?

What helps and what hinders partnership working?

Although the evidence on outcomes is limited, there is a growing body of literature on what partnerships themselves and other local stakeholders feel help to develop interagency relationships. Typically, this literature is much stronger on the pre-existing conditions for successful partnership and on the factors that should exist in an ideal scenario than it is on what to do if this is not the case in your area. Put simply, there is a slightly simplistic tendency to assume that issues such as trust and reciprocity are fundamental, without necessarily exploring how best to proceed if partner agencies in your area cannot stand each other and never speak!

This overly optimistic element of the literature aside, much of the existing evidence – both from formal research and from practical experience of working in interagency settings – tends to be summarised in a series of frameworks. Often very accessible and succinct, these run the risk of trying to reduce a much more complex reality down into a series of simple 'rules', but do provide a helpful checklist against which to compare current relationships. Three prominent examples are set in Boxes 2.4 to 2.6, and frontline practitioners and/or managers may wish to follow these up in more detail with a view to using them to understand their own local partnerships in more depth.

Box 2.4: The Partnership Assessment Tool

Developed through ongoing research by the former Nuffield Institute at the University of Leeds, the Partnership Assessment Tool (PAT) provides an opportunity for a routine 'health check' of local partnerships, helps to identify areas of potential conflict and provides a developmental framework for establishing a healthy and effective partnership.

Based on six partnership principles, PAT supports local partners to rate their achievement against various key criteria, providing a quick and easy means of analysing results and identifying issues that require further work. The six key principles that PAT explores are the extent to which partners:

* recognise and accept the need for partnership
* develop clarity and realism of purpose
* ensure commitment and ownership
* develop and maintain trust
* create clear and robust partnership arrangements
* monitor, measure and learn.

—

Available online via the Department for Communities and Local Government, PAT is probably the best known and most widely used of such tools (Hardy et al, 2003).

Box 2.5: The Working Partnership

Developed by the former Health Development Agency (since merged into the National Institute for Health and Clinical Excellence), the Working Partnership is a boxed set of documents that provide a short overview assessment of any given interagency partnership, a more in-depth assessment to review strengths and areas for improvement, and guidance on approaches to ensuring continuous improvement. In particular, the tool focuses on six key elements of good practice in partnership working:

- *leadership* (including shared vision, ownership and commitment, and recognition of key external relationships);
- *organisation* (including public participation, flexible working arrangements, transparent management and communication);
- *strategy* (including strategic development, information and evaluation and action and review);
- *learning* (including valuing people, developing knowledge and skills and supporting innovation);
- *resources* (including building social capital, pooling financial resources and using information and technology appropriately);
- *programmes* (developing coordinated programmes and integrated services through joint planning, focused delivery and monitoring and review).

Source: Markwell et al (2003)

Box 2.6: The Partnership Readiness Framework

Developed by Greig and Poxton (2001), the Partnership Readiness Framework highlights the key building blocks of successful partnership:

- building and agreeing shared values and principles with a vision of how life should be for people who use services;
- agreeing specific policy shifts that the partnership arrangements are designed to achieve;
- being prepared to explore new service options and not be tied too closely to existing services or providers;
- being clear about what aspects of service and activity are inside and outside the boundaries of the partnership arrangements;
- being clear about organisational roles in terms of responsibilities for and relationships between commissioning, purchasing and providing;
- identifying agreed resource pools and putting to one side unresolved historical disagreements;
- ensuring effective leadership, including senior level commitment to the partnership agenda;
- providing sufficient partnership development capacity rather than it being a small and marginalised part of everyone's role;
- developing and sustaining good personal relationships, creating opportunities and incentives for key players to nurture these relationships in order to promote mutual trust.

Using key frameworks in practice

Although such frameworks are inevitably simple in their approach, they do offer a useful short-hand way of trying to understand what helps and what hinders effective partnership working. When used as the authors intended, moreover, they become more of a way of assessing current relationships, understanding what it is possible to achieve in the current context and identifying areas that require further work. Furthermore, while there is a danger that they can seem over-simplistic, many of the factors that they identify seem to reflect what local managers and practitioners experience when trying to work together more effectively. At their best, therefore, such tools can help to make sense of the barriers that frontline partnerships experience, as well as offering potential insight into what needs to happen next and cautioning of the need to keep our partnership aspirations realistic. As an example of this, Box 2.7 cites some anonymised but real-life case studies of the way in which such frameworks can add value to attempts to develop more effective partnerships.

Box 2.7: Using relevant tools in practice

In one health and social care community, partners from local mental health services used the Partnership Readiness Framework to explore the extent to which local services were ready for the large-scale changes that they were planning. After using this tool, the partnership decided instead that local services were actually in the process of overcoming a long-standing legacy of mistrust and poor communication, and that an approach that identified some earlier and easier 'quick wins' would be a helpful way of rebuilding trust and developing momentum for the future.

In another area, the Working Partnership helped local partners to celebrate the progress they had made together in developing a more trusting long-term relationship, but also identified areas on which partners needed to focus if future progress was to be made.

When reorganising primary care services in 2006, the Department of Health sought to scrutinise proposals for new PCTs in terms of the implications of the changes for health and local government partnerships. In doing so, the factors identified by the PAT were recommended as a way of assessing local proposals and judging the likely success of the relationships that these new organisational boundaries implied.

Limits of structural change

If we still know relatively little about what works when it comes to health and social care partnerships, we have learned some key lessons about what does not work (see below for further discussion). In particular, there is growing evidence to suggest that structural change – by itself – is not an effective means of achieving more effective partnerships or better outcomes for the people who use services. While this is discussed in more detail in another book in this series by Peck and Dickinson (*Managing and leading in inter-agency settings*), the literature on structural change and reorganisation suggests that:

- structural change alone rarely achieves its stated objectives;
- in addition to stated drivers for the merger, there are usually unstated drivers (such as addressing managerial or financial deficits and responding to local or national politics);
- the economic benefits are modest at best, and may be out-weighed by unanticipated direct costs and unintended negative consequences (such as a decline in productivity and morale);
- senior management time is often focused on the process of merger, and this can stall positive service development for at least 18 months (if not longer);
- the after-effects of mergers can continue for many years after the change has taken place.

(See, for example, Craig and Manthorpe, 1999; Fulop et al, 2002, 2005; Field and Peck, 2003; SSI/Audit Commission, 2004; Peck and Freeman, 2005.)

On many occasions, of course, there can be a tendency for policy makers seeking to develop and improve public services to look to the private sector for successful models and approaches. In the case of structural change, however, the evidence from private sector mergers and acquisitions is positively alarming. As Field and Peck (2003, p 743) have demonstrated, 'one of the key messages in the literature on [private sector] mergers is that they have happened at an astonishing pace despite the fact that they do not appear to be beneficial when judged

—

on economic criteria'. According to one source, for instance, 54% of acquisitions were regarded as failures (Coopers & Lybrand, 1993). Consequently, many commercial organisations considering mergers have increasingly begun to pay attention to the human (cultural) factors involved in this process, rather than simply trying to create better results by changing structures (see below for further discussion).

Despite the overwhelming evidence about the limits of structural change, it seems more than a little ironic to note that this still seems to be a favourite tactic of national policy makers – particularly in the NHS. As Walshe (2003) has demonstrated, the NHS has been reorganised on an almost constant basis for the past two decades or so, with four main impacts:

- The proposed benefits of each reform are never achieved in practice, as the system has always been reorganised again before any meaningful evaluation can take place.
- Significant resources (both financial and human) are wasted (through the diversion of senior management time, new offices, new letterheads, new signs etc).
- The process of reform is commonly circular, with similar structures and solutions re-emerging over time.
- Constant change ironically makes the system highly change-resistant, as staff become increasingly cynical and short-term in their focus.

The overall result, as Walshe suggests in a vivid and depressingly accurate summary (2003, p 108), is that the NHS is 'an organizational shantytown in which structures and systems are cobbled together or thrown up hastily in the knowledge that they will be torn down in due course'. At various stages in recent years, of course, structural change has also been put forward as a potential solution to the problematic nature of the health and social care divide, with the care trust model (see Glasby and Peck, 2003) probably the most visible example of this approach. Thus, despite current commitments to notions of 'evidence-based policy' (see below for further discussion), the temptation of an apparently quick and bold structural solution seems almost too much to resist, and the risk is that we end up damaging existing health and social care partnerships in the name of trying to support and improve them. This is perhaps best captured by Hudson (2002, p 82), who observes that:

> [In the case of care trusts], there remains a strong political commitment to an untried model. In the light of the emphasis normally placed by the Department of Health on evidence based approaches to policy and practice, this is perhaps a surprising turn of events.

As something of an aside, there is also now a growing literature on how best to manage and lead organisations during periods of merger and structural change. While this is explored in more detail in the book by Peck and Dickinson in this series (*Managing and leading in inter-agency settings*), Box 2.8 below summarises some of the key messages from a review of this literature.

Box 2.8: Lessons from the literature on managing organisations during structural change

There are four distinct time periods within the merger process, with different approaches and management behaviour required in each different phase.

Prior to merger, it is important to assess the culture of each of the merging organisations and to use this knowledge as part of a careful strategy for highlighting and recognising the differences between the organisations.

Having decided to merge, managers and leaders should communicate a vision that sets out the purpose of changes and do this in an open and participatory manner.

During merger, key practical steps include providing practical and emotional support for staff, making human resources (HR) the main issue, communicating relentlessly, setting up clear transitional structures to guide and implement the merger, and helping staff to understand the implications of change.

> *After merger,* it is important to monitor and evaluate the impact of the change for at least three years – both in relation to the original objectives and using other measures such as staff attitudes and service user/carer satisfaction.
>
> *Source:* Dickinson et al (2006)

Whose fault is this lack of evidence?

As a post-script to this chapter, it is important to think through whose fault this situation may be. Is it the politicians (who might be accused of developing policy in advance of the evidence and jumping on the 'partnership bandwagon')? Is it the academics (who have arguably been slow to respond to the partnership agenda)? Is it frontline services (who have perhaps understandably tended to focus more on implementing change than on evaluating its longer-term impact)? In one sense, the answer is probably that all these groups and factors have contributed to our lack of knowledge about the impact of partnership working. And yet, there is probably a fourth culprit as well – the nature of 'evidence' itself.

Although this may sound strange initially, traditional notions of 'evidence-based practice' have often been dominated by formal research and, in health and social care, by approaches associated with medicine and with science (that is, by quantitative research and by very formal and precise methods known as randomised controlled trials and systematic reviews). As a result, current debates about 'the evidence' often tend to focus only on very selective understandings of what should constitute valid evidence, and a large number of dissenting voices are often overlooked. While this is discussed in more detail elsewhere (see, for example, Rycroft-Malone et al, 2004; Glasby and Beresford, 2006; Glasby et al, 2007), a good example of this is the systematic reviews common in some parts of the NHS, which initially identify several thousand studies, exclude all but a very small number of quantitative studies, then conclude that there is very little research available!

Although clearly a caricature of a much more complex issue, there do seem to be clear instances in both health and social care where a narrow focus on very traditional notions of what constitutes valid evidence can lead to a very limited insight into the issues at stake (and the issue of health and social care partnerships may well be an example of this). As a result, it is possible that we may understand more about the nature and impact of partnerships if we adopt a different approach to understanding 'what works'. While this is a broader issue than can be dealt with in full here, possible examples include:

- Focusing not on 'what works' so much as on 'what does not work'. While we still know relatively little about the outcomes of partnership working, there is significant evidence of the limitations of single agency approaches. Instead of waiting for 'the evidence' before implementing new ways of working, therefore, an important step forward would be to decide what does not work in the current system, do something different and test out whether this works better (essentially a form of learning 'what works' by doing and reflecting). Inevitably, this might mean a very different role for those national bodies currently responsible for improving health and social care services and for disseminating good practice.

- Basing future decisions not just on what formal research has to tell us, but also on what we believe we have learned from previous changes and from current ways of working (essentially a move away from 'evidence-based practice' to a notion of 'practice-based evidence').

- Expanding traditional (often very medically dominated) notions of evidence to include other ways of knowing the world, such as the lived experience of users and carers, and the tacit knowledge of frontline practitioners (essentially a move away from traditional 'evidence-based practice' to a broader, more inclusive notion of 'knowledge-based practice').

—

Thus, the overall result of this discussion is that we do not yet know what impact partnership working has, for whom or under what circumstances. However, the reality is that we are probably unlikely to know this with any certainty for some time (if ever). As a result, the best way forward in the short term may be for health and social care practitioners and their organisations to be clear about what they are trying to achieve by working together, and to build in appropriate critical reflection and evaluation to enable them to learn as they go along. (In many ways, this builds on a broader theoretical approach known as 'realistic evaluation', and Chapter 4 provides a more detailed summary of the key concepts and frameworks that this entails.) While such an approach may not always seem very convincing to a busy manager or a national policy maker under pressure to ensure that their next policy is 'evidence-based', this nevertheless seems a more constructive way forward than arguing that we cannot do anything because we do not have enough 'evidence'.

Reflective exercises

1. Reflecting on recent experiences of working with someone from a different organisational or professional background, what (if anything) were you able to achieve together that you could not have done on your own? Where this relationship went well, what were the key underlying success factors? Where it went badly, what were the key barriers that prevented progress? After sharing these reflections with other colleagues, what does this start to tell you about what helps and hinders partnership working?

2. Using PAT, the Working Partnership or the Partnership Readiness Framework above, how successful do current local partnerships appear, and what practical recommendations could you make to improve local interagency collaboration?

---

3. Reflecting on a local partnership, how ready for partnership working were local partners, and on which key areas of the relationship do they need to do further development work?

4. For any given case study partnership (for example, a care trust, a pooled budget or a joint appointment), how could you go about evaluating the success of the partnership? In particular, what was the partnership designed to achieve, how would you know if it had been successful, and what might have happened anyway had the partnership not been in place?

Further reading and resources

For key research studies on health and social care (and broader) partnerships, see the national evaluations of partnership initiatives, such as:

- the Children's Fund (Edwards et al, 2006)
- children's trusts (University of East Anglia, 2007)
- the Health Act flexibilities (Glendinning et al, 2002b)
- HAZs (Barnes et al, 2005)
- intermediate care (Godfrey et al, 2005; Barton et al, 2006)
- LAAs (ODPM, 2005a, 2007)
- LSPs (ODPM and Department for Transport, 2006)
- Sure Start (www.ness.bbk.ac.uk)

At a more local level, a particularly important insight is provided by Peck et al's (2002) innovative study of health and social care partnerships in Somerset. At the time, this was the first integrated health and social care organisation outside Northern Ireland, and this, coupled with Somerset's brave decision to commission and publicise an evaluation, is a crucial source of evidence (albeit one that, as discussed above, is open to multiple interpretations).

For a critical and more theoretical summary of the limitations of current approaches to evaluating partnerships, see Helen Dickinson's book in this current series (*Evaluating outcomes in health and social care*), as well as her (2006) article on 'The evaluation of health and social care partnerships'.

See Dickinson et al (2006) for a discussion of the research evidence on *Leadership in organisational transition*.

For a practical online tool for evaluating the outcome of health and social care partnerships see the Partnership Outcomes Evaluation Toolkit (POET), developed by the Health Services Management Centre and available via www.hsmc.bham.ac.uk

—

3

Hot topics and emerging issues

Having explored key concepts and summarised key research findings, this chapter explores a series of current tensions in the relationship between health, social care and other partners, including:

- Can effective partnerships ever be 'forced' by central policy?
- How can health and social care work with each other while also trying to work with broader partners?
- How do we ensure accountability and what happens when money is involved?
- How can we be responsible for services delegated to partner agencies?
- How do we ensure that partnerships remain focused on what service users and patients want?
- Do partnerships lead to better outcomes, is it worth it and how can we tell?

Sadly, with the lack of evidence described in Chapter 2, it is hard to be definitive about many (if any) of these questions. In many ways, therefore, the issues explored below represent a very good example of areas in which lessons learned the hard way in frontline policy and practice are far ahead of the current evidence base from formal research. However, the discussion below is an attempt to draw together – from various sources – what we already know about such 'hot topics', and to pose a series of additional challenges for frontline practitioners and services seeking to develop more effective partnerships to reflect on.

Legal duties and 'forced' partnerships

While much of the literature on effective partnership working emphasises issues such as trust, reciprocity, autonomy and shared vision, there are many examples of situations in which partners have no choice but to work in partnership. At a national level, statutes such as the Health Act (1999), the Children Act (2004) and the Local Government and Public Involvement in Health Act (2007) set out various duties to cooperate and to work in partnership. However, such commitments are often very vague, and are typically more symbolic than practical when it comes to ensuring effective partnerships at a local level. Although it is a slightly tongue-in-cheek example, what would happen to a health and social care community that was deemed to be breaking its statutory obligations to work in partnership? How would we identify such a breach of the law, prove the accusation and hold the agencies concerned to account? In any case, what do such duties actually mean in practice, and at what stage in a problematic relationship do we decide that such legal duties are not being discharged? Even if all these questions were answered, what would happen in practice to the chief executives of each partner agency? As some policy commentators suggest in private, when the first fine is levied or the first senior manager 'named and shamed' for failure to collaborate across agency boundaries, then such legal duties may be perceived as having more 'teeth' than at present (personal communications).

In practice, of course, such legal provisions send out a potentially powerful symbolic message about the importance that policy makers attach to partnership working – by devising duties of partnership, those who make our laws are effectively sending a very clear and welcome signal that not working together is not an option and will not be tolerated. However, moving from a general symbolic message such as this to implementing and supporting lasting change at local level is a more complex and fraught process. While these issues are discussed in much more detail in the broader literature on policy making (see, for example, Hill, 2004; Buse et al, 2005; Baggott, 2007), recent partnership policies have been designed in very different ways with very different underlying assumptions about what motivates frontline practitioners and about what changes behaviour at ground level.

At its most extreme, this debate often focuses on the extent to which it is either possible or desirable to compel practitioners and local organisations to work together (for a discussion of so-called *mandated collaboration* see Rodríguez et al, 2007). A good example of this issue is the debate around how best to reduce the number of people whose stay in hospital is delayed due to problems in the discharge process. While hospital discharge has long been a problematic area of policy and practice (for a summary, see Glasby, 2003), it became an increasing policy priority from 2000 onwards following government concerns that delays attributed to social care may be jeopardising commitments around NHS waiting times. Following the investment of additional money, the main response from policy makers in England was the controversial 2003 Community Care (Delayed Discharges etc) Act, which introduced a system of 'cross-charging' (subsequently described as a system of 'reimbursement').

From the beginning, such a policy divided commentators. While some felt that this was an overly simplistic approach that unfairly penalised social care for what was essentially an interagency issue, others claimed that delaying hospital discharge due to delays in arranging or funding social care services was unacceptable and had to be tackled. In particular, much of the discussion centred on the extent to which such an apparently punitive approach was the best way of promoting the long-term interagency relationships required to tackle the root of the problem. As is often the case, much of the most heated debate took place before the policy came into force, and the clumsy way in which the policy was initially handled did much to increase the tension (Henwood, 2006). However, following a change in emphasis, the provision of an additional grant and the support of a government Change Agent Team, many health and social care communities were nevertheless able to develop much more joint and positive approaches, using the reimbursement legislation as a springboard from which to develop a more genuinely multiagency response. Despite this, doubts remain about the extent to which a policy based ultimately on blaming and 'fining' one 'partner' for perceived under-performance is the best way of developing effective partnerships (see Box 3.1).

—

Box 3.1: Reimbursement and hospital discharge as an example of 'forced' partnership

As Henwood (2006) explains, the 2003 Community Care (Delayed Discharges etc) Act introduces a system whereby NHS bodies must notify social services of a patient's likely need for community care services (a Section 2 notification). There is a defined timescale (at least three days) for social services to complete the individual's assessment and provide appropriate social care services. A second notice (a Section 5 notification) follows completion of a multidisciplinary assessment and gives notice of the proposed day of discharge (minimum of 24 hours notice). A reimbursement charge of £100 per day (£120 per day in London/the South East) is paid by social services to the acute trust if the fact of social services not having met their obligations is the sole reason for the delay in discharge from hospital. NHS bodies have to make both of the notifications to social services if a claim for reimbursement is to be triggered. Liability for payment begins on the day after the three days of the assessment notification, or the day after the proposed discharge date, whichever is later.

As soon as this policy was announced, there were immediate concerns that this would encourage premature discharge and emergency readmission, that it would damage existing relationships between health and social care and that it unfairly penalised one partner for a genuinely whole systems problem. In contrast, others rightly argued that hospital was an inappropriate place for older people in particular to be when they no longer needed the services provided there, and that any policy that encouraged swift discharge and a more effective use of scarce resources was to be welcomed.

Following the implementation of the new system, delays did initially fall (although they had already been falling before the new policy and the rate of reduction now seems to have levelled off somewhat). In the main, health and social care communities have typically worked hard to ensure that the 'horror stories' predicted by some commentators have not materialised, and many have negotiated a system whereby both partners invest in rehabilitative services, with no charges payable until the level of the 'fines' amassed exceeds the amount that social care has invested up-front in new services. However, concerns remain that such a policy may not be the best way of securing long-term change and that the introduction of such financial incentives may have unintended consequences (for example, on the risk of premature discharge, on the rate of care home admissions from hospital and/or on the rate of emergency hospital readmissions).

For a full discussion of these issues, see accounts by CSCI (2004, 2005), Glasby (2003) and Henwood (2004, 2006).

More than misquoting a popular saying, therefore, it seems as though you can lead health and social care partners to water, and probably even make them drink. Whether or not you can use the same tactics to make them agree how to make best use of the scarce water at their disposal (and to continue both drinking and cooperating when you stop monitoring them in this way) remains open to question.

In an important contribution to this debate, Rodríguez et al (2007) argue that 'mandated collaboration' involves three different types of governance:

- bureaucratic mechanisms (such as the introduction of new rules and regulations);
- new incentives to encourage partners to alter previous behaviour;
- interaction between partners to aid mutual understanding.

Returning to the earlier discussion about different ways of organising public services (see Chapter 1), Rodríguez et al see these approaches as representative of the three organisational types explored in Box 1.2:

- hierarchical approaches to compel joint working;
- market-based approaches to provide new incentives;

- network-based approaches to enable more informal interaction, shared values and cooperation.

According to this analysis, many attempts at 'forced partnership' may fail if they concentrate solely on mandating the partnership, without sufficient rules, incentives or interaction to make the policy work. Applying this to the discussion of reimbursement above, initial policy certainly seems to have been guilty of this approach, with subsequent attempts to implement the policy enjoying more success as a result of a more nuanced blend of hierarchy, market and network (for a discussion of the need for 'requisite variety' see also Peck and 6, 2006).

Of course, the extent to which it is possible to create 'forced' partnerships is actually an outward manifestation of a deeper issue: how best to encourage change in public services. Again, this is discussed in more detail in the policy literature. However, our own belief is that previous policies have attempted to change behaviour at the front line in at least three different ways:

- by 'making' people behave differently (through the use of legislation or mechanisms such as reimbursement above);
- by the 'power of ideas' (exhorting people to behave differently and appealing to rational debate about the best way forward);
- by 'structural change' (see Chapter 2 for a critique of our tendency to rely on this approach in the NHS in particular).

For any given social issue and policy response, a mix of these approaches may be required in practice (and the nature of that balance will change according to the current context, the nature of the issue and the perceived urgency of the issues at stake). However, we believe that a more powerful way of changing practice is to *change accountabilities*, and that the other approaches summarised above often get used in the short term only as a more superficial and simplistic proxy. It is for this reason, we would argue, that repeated NHS reorganisation seems to have little effect (although this looks like and is often justified in terms of changing accountabilities, it typically happens so frequently and focuses so much on structural change that the underlying accountabilities remain the same). It is also for this reason that social care policies such as direct payments and individual budgets seem so exciting and potentially transformative (as they fundamentally alter the accountability between services and welfare professionals on the one hand, and people who use services on the other – for an introduction to direct payments see Glasby and Littlechild, 2002). We are also reminded of an NHS proposal to change the way in which hospital doctors are remunerated, basing a proportion of pay on patient satisfaction (*Health Service Journal*, 2006; Britnell, 2007). While this latter proposal is controversial, one of the reasons why it would arouse such strong feelings if ever implemented is that it starts to ask doctors to whom they feel accountable – their Royal College, their peers, their chief executive or their patients?

In a partnership context, it is hard to know how managers and policy makers could think about changing accountabilities in order to support more effective partnership working. Perhaps if there was a single set of targets for each health and social care community (with individual agencies held to account for the performance of all agencies across the whole system), this might make practitioners and managers feel more accountable to each other and to national policy makers for the overall performance of the system (not just their individual component part)? Perhaps a system of performance-related pay and career progression based in part on feedback from other professions and organisations could begin to change interprofessional behaviour? Perhaps extending direct payments and individual budgets from social care to the NHS would enable service users to decide how best to integrate services to meet their own health and social care needs? Whether readers agree or disagree with such approaches (and whether or not they are ever implemented in practice), we believe that a deeper debate about to whom health and social care practitioners feel accountable is a more constructive way forward than simply discussing whether or not 'forced partnerships' are effective.

Working with broader partners

Although previous policy and literature has tended to focus on the health and social care divide as one of the main barriers to more effective services for people with cross-cutting needs, there has been a more recent recognition of the need to work with broader partners and more universal services. In England, services for children and for adults are now increasingly separate, with each tasked with delivering a series of outcomes on behalf of people who use services (see Box 3.2). However, if health and social care really are to deliver these challenging outcomes, then working with each other will not be enough – many of the outcomes concerned are so broad and so complex to achieve that there will need to be a coordinated and concerted effort from a range of stakeholders across the public, private and voluntary sectors. Although it is hard to disagree with a commitment to ensuring that children are able to make a positive contribution or that a frail older person enjoys greater economic well-being, delivering this in practice will probably require the input of a large number of agencies, including the NHS, the full range of local government services and many more potential partners besides (see, for example, Manthorpe et al, 2006). While this is a laudable goal, it remains very challenging for frontline agencies to deliver in practice, particularly in a policy context where so many of the relevant targets, legal frameworks and financial incentives seem to encourage single agency approaches. In many ways, the same is also true of current imperatives to develop a more preventative approach and to provide better support for people with long-term conditions (DH, 2006) – again, delivering these bold aspirations will require a range of agencies (and potentially very uneasy bedfellows) coming together to make this happen in practice.

Box 3.2: Outcomes for children and for adults

In children's services, partners are tasked with ensuring that children and young people (HM Treasury, 2003):

- are healthy
- stay safe
- are able to enjoy and achieve
- make a positive contribution
- experience economic well-being.

In adult services, proposed outcomes include (DH, 2006):

- improved health and emotional well-being
- improved quality of life
- making a positive contribution
- choice and control
- freedom from discrimination
- economic well-being
- personal dignity.

As a practical example of the issues at stake, a national workshop commissioned by the Valuing People Support Team brought together a number of key national stakeholders to explore the future of services for people with learning difficulties (Glasby, 2004). This included an invited audience of people with learning difficulties, their carers, voluntary organisations, academics and government departments (including health and social care, local government and education). In particular, participants were very clear that people with learning difficulties want the same things and should have the same rights to a good life as everyone else (see Figures 3.1 and 3.2). Indeed, a group of people with learning difficulties asked to start the workshop summarised this in terms of three key things that they wanted from services and from life more generally:

- *Money*, including financial independence, choosing where you live and who supports you, and being able to enjoy fun things like shopping and holidays.
- *Food*, including access to information to make decisions about healthy lifestyles as well as the ability to make choices about everyday things like what you eat, where you live and what you wear.

Figure 3.1: What people with learning disabilities want and need

Family carers

Information

Planning for life

Health

A place to live

Keeping safe

Leisure and social activities

Speaking up

Friendships and relationships

Work

Support in daily living

Learning

Money

Source: Greig (2000), quoted in Glasby (2004)

- *Sex and relationships*, including friends and relationships, the right to a social life and a private life, the right to have sexual relationships and to get married, and having children and being a family.

While these were in some ways very modest requests, traditional health and social care services continue to struggle to provide even these basic human needs on behalf of people with learning difficulties. In part, participants argued, this is because we have seen the needs of people with learning difficulties as being somehow specialist in nature, and have tried to meet them through (often segregated) health and social services. However, many people present questioned the rationale

Figure 3.2: Services involved (or not) in meeting the aspirations of people with learning difficulties

Source: Greig (2000), quoted in Glasby (2004)

for this – if someone has a need for education, meaningful leisure opportunities and decent housing, then surely these needs should be met through existing education, leisure and housing services, not through specialist health and social care? Although this makes perfect sense, the problem is that we have inherited a system in which these much broader, supposedly more universal services have been designed and run without people with learning difficulties in mind, and that current targets often fail to support local organisations to work across departmental boundaries to meet the needs of groups such as people with learning difficulties. While all present wanted to challenge and change this, doing it in practice remained problematic with few easy answers.

Essentially, therefore, documents such as *Valuing People*, *Our health, our care, our say* and *Every Child Matters* (DH, 2001, 2006; HM Treasury, 2003) ask health and social care to work with each other, while also working with broader, more universal services. At the same time, many of these policy documents arguably fail to establish in full the structures and the mechanisms needed to deliver this vision in practice, and frontline services consistently report that they feel progress is hindered by:

- a lack of incentives for broader partners to focus on the needs of people with health and social care needs;
- a lack of shared history, joint ownership or cultural fit between health and social care on the one hand, and broader partners on the other – for all that the health and social care divide is problematic, it remains one of life's ironies that health and social care often seem to have so much more in common with each other than social care does with other local authority services;
- the difficulty in bringing together services that target their resources on specific groups with services that offer a (supposedly) universal service for all.

While progress is slowly being made on these issues at a national and a local level, it remains difficult to be confident that such tensions can be resolved in the short term.

Accountability and risk

In Chapter 1, we suggested that partnership working has traditionally been seen as a 'good thing', but that there has been more recent recognition of some of the negatives associated with partnerships (see, for example, Box 1.9). In many ways, this is part of a more recent reaction against partnerships, in which frontline services and practitioners are (perhaps rightly) starting to adopt what we see as a more sceptical approach. In many ways this trend is illustrated by growing concerns about issues of risk and accountability, and by a 2005 report published by the Audit Commission, *Governing partnerships*. According to the latter, partnerships can be crucial in delivering improvements in people's quality of life, but can also bring risks as well as opportunities. In particular, partnerships may not always deliver value for money (given the direct and indirect costs associated), while the complexity and ambiguity that partnership working entails can 'generate confusion and weaken accountability' (p 2). In addition, the Commission found that areas such as leadership, decision making, scrutiny and risk management were all under-developed in partnerships. Above all, 'local public bodies should be much more constructively critical about this form of working: it may not be the best solution in every case' (Audit Commission, 2005, p 2).

While these issues are discussed in more detail by Glasby and Peck (2006) and in the book on leadership in this series (*Managing and leading in inter-agency settings*, by Peck and Dickinson), current and recent partnerships do seem increasingly concerned to be clear about their accountabilities and about what happens when money is 'involved. In many ways, this is entirely right and proper, and no one would presumably argue against greater transparency about such important issues. However, quite how to achieve this in practice remains problematic, and opinions vary as to the best way forward. While the Audit Commission (2005) emphasises the need for 'partnership agreements' as a means of ensuring good governance, we have a slightly different take on the issues (for a more detailed analysis see Glasby and Peck, 2006). According to our earlier discussion about hierarchies, markets and networks (see Chapter 1), some would argue that a crucial feature of partnerships is the extent to which they enable individual organisations to retain the right of exit (which is very different to a market-based contract, for example). Playing devil's advocate somewhat, any partner agencies that need very detailed legal agreement about respective roles and responsibilities would surely be better off signing a formal contract, rather than opting for the more informal and flexible approach that a partnership entails. Presumably for some partners it is exactly this flexibility and this right of exit that makes partnership an attractive proposition in the first place, and subsequent governance arrangements need to strike an appropriate balance between protection, probity, room for manoeuvre and clarity of roles and responsibilities. As a very rough rule of thumb (and only slightly tongue in cheek), it has been suggested that any partnership that needs an agreement that is more than a few pages long is probably not really a partnership in the first place.

Working through partner agencies

Closely linked to issues of risk and accountability is a further question about how best to ensure that individual agencies continue to meet their moral and legal obligations once they have delegated day-to-day responsibility for delivering services to a partner agency. It was precisely this issue that lay at the heart of the formal investigation in Cornwall, with inspectors (Healthcare Commission/CSCI, 2006, p 7) arguing that services delivered via a so-called NHS 'partnership' trust had very little involvement from social care at all and that relationships between the trust and the county council were poor (for a summary of some of the key partnership-related findings see Box 3.3).

Box 3.3: Findings from an investigation into services for people with learning difficulties in Cornwall

In 2006, a joint investigation into the provision of services for people with learning difficulties at Cornwall Partnership NHS Trust found evidence of institutional abuse, poor practice and a lack of appropriate leadership.

In addition, inspectors found that:

- PCT commissioning of services was inadequate with insufficient monitoring.
- 'Working relationships between the trust and Cornwall County Council have been poor for a considerable time'.

- 'Services for people with learning disabilities were not transferred to social services, following the closure of long stay hospitals, as they were in other parts of the UK'.
- 'Social services have had little involvement in the care provided by the trust'.
- Learning disability services were marginalised, both within the trust itself (which focused primarily on mental health services) and by the strategic health authority.

Source: Healthcare Commission/CSCI (2006, p 7)

Responding to this dilemma is difficult, and many organisations find it hard to get the balance right between giving a lead partner the flexibility to deliver on joint priorities while at the same time remaining sufficiently involved to be able both to support and to scrutinise that partner. All too often, this seems to result in a situation where the original partner either delegates formal responsibilities (yet does not really trust the other partner to deliver), or sees any functions it has delegated as 'somebody else's problem' and actively disengages. To guard against these dangers, mechanisms such as health scrutiny may have a key role to play, with the local authority able to use its powers to promote the well-being of the local area in order to examine the quality of various health services (see, for example, www.cfps.org.uk/health). Where health and social care are increasingly working together, one option would be to focus the work of the health scrutiny committee on an area of joint work, using this process not so much to hold the NHS to account, but rather to act as a critical friend with regard to existing partnerships and joint services. Another approach explored by some of the early care trusts was to ring-fence initial social care budgets and to stipulate that any major reconfiguration of social care services had to be agreed by the council. This was initially put in place for a few years as a way of gradually building trust and confidence in the partnership from all parties, with a view to revisiting and potentially removing such safeguards once all local partners were confident in the ability of the care trust to deliver on a joint agenda (for a further discussion of care trusts, see Glasby and Peck, 2003).

Staying focused on service users

Part of the problem with the current policy context is that partnerships are now so widespread that it is hard to continue to see them as a means to an end. This is a consistent theme throughout this book, and is explored in more detail in Chapter 4. However, opinion is divided as to whether partnership working is a 'good thing' from the perspective of people who use services. While some claim that partnerships are a potentially helpful way of responding to the needs of service users and to their desire for more coordinated, holistic services, others see greater partnership working as leading to reduced choice and a greater concentration of power in favour of services rather than of service users. A good example here is provided by current debates in mental health services, with some commentators arguing that the integration of health and social care runs the risk of denying service users access to more social, non-medical alternatives to traditional psychiatric approaches (see Box 3.4). Similarly, greater collaboration between services such as health and social care offers the potential of more coordinated, better resourced and more meaningful approaches to user and patient involvement, while at the same time running the risk of reducing sources of support and opportunities to voice their concerns should service users be dissatisfied with current services.

Box 3.4: Ambiguities of partnership working from a user perspective: the case of mental health services

Potential advantages of partnership (in theory):

- single point of entry
- less sense of being passed 'from pillar to post'
- more holistic response to need
- greater coordination of support
- broader range of services.

Potential disadvantages:

- scope for medical model to dominate other perspectives
- potential for more social alternatives to be overshadowed by psychiatric approaches
- less chance for one partner to advocate on behalf of users with the other partner
- possible loss of local services as the partnership rationalises its provision
- having one point of contact can give users nowhere else to go if this attempt to contact services does not work as well as it should
- concerns about a loss of key relationships with staff and about potential change in use of local buildings.

Source: Personal communications, service users receiving support from partnership trusts

In addition to these issues, Skelcher et al (2004) raise a series of challenges about the threats that partnerships can pose to local democracy. In a series of research studies and commentaries, they argue that partnerships can be a flexible vehicle by which entrepreneurial managers exercise greater discretion over local services and that partnerships often engage the public and service users in their work. However, decision makers on partnership boards are typically public service managers, and the subsequent partnership can bypass traditional forms of local democracy and accountability (that is, elected members and local councils). Partnerships also have very different and variable approaches to issues such as public access, transparency and openness, with standards typically falling below accepted good practice. As part of this debate, Skelcher et al (2004) have developed a Governance Assessment Tool (see Box 3.5) that partnerships can use to assess the extent to which they conform to current good practice standards around such issues of accountability and probity.

Box 3.5: Governance Assessment Tool

Public accessibility

1. Are meetings of the board advertised?
2. Are meetings of the board open to the press and public?
3. Are the public entitled to see reports considered by the board?
4. Are the reports that the board will consider available for the public to consult prior to the meeting?
5. Are the public entitled to see minutes of board meetings?
6. Is there an annual general meeting that the public can attend?

Internal governance

1. Does the partnership have a memorandum of association or other document defining its role and powers?
2. Does the partnership have a written constitution or set of standing orders defining how it will conduct its business at meetings?
3. Is membership for a limited period of time? If so, how long?
4. Does a quorum apply at board meetings? If so, what is it?
5. Are written minutes of board meetings produced?
6. Are there allowances or other payments for members? If so, how much?

Member conduct

1. Is there a code of conduct to regulate the behaviour of members at board meetings?
2. If there is a code, are board members required to agree to be bound by it?
3. Is there a register in which board members detail their financial and other interests? If so, is this compulsory? And is it open for public inspection?
4. Is there a system for declaring conflicts of interest at meetings? If so, what is the procedure and where is it set down?

5. Is there a procedure for ensuring that members declaring conflicts of interest take no part in the decision? If so, what is the procedure and where is it set down?

Accountability

1. Does the partnership have to prepare an annual report? If yes, is this a public document?
2. Does the partnership have to prepare an annual budget? If yes, is this a public document?
3. Does the partnership have to prepare annual accounts? If yes, is this a public document?
4. Is the partnership subject to external audit?
5. Is the partnership subject to external inspection?
6. Is there a complaints process available to citizens or service users?
7. Is the partnership under the jurisdiction of an ombudsman or inspectorate?
8. Is the partnership required to meet targets agreed with any other bodies?
9. Does the partnership make a formal report to any other bodies (including the member organisations)?
10. Can members be recalled by their nominating bodies?

Source: Skelcher et al (2004); for further information, see www.inlogov.bham.ac.uk/research/esrcpartnership.htm

Helpful though this tool is as a means of thinking through governance issues, it does tend to assume that current approaches in local government represent a gold standard against which other ways of delivering services should be judged. While this may be true in terms of the formal rules that govern conduct and access in local government, the reality is arguably a system in which such theoretical rights become less meaningful as a result of difficulties that many members of the public face when seeking to understanding and engage with the culture and bureaucracy of many local authorities. Although the NHS is often portrayed as having a 'democratic deficit', a more accurate description would be to say that social care is accountable to locally elected politicians, while the NHS is accountable nationally to a Secretary of State who is appointed by the democratically elected government of the day. With low turnouts in recent local elections, moreover, it is at least debatable as to whether the Secretary of State or the local councillor has a greater democratic mandate.

Ultimately, therefore, what is at stake here may be two alternative visions of the future:

• Will two already large, powerful and frequently inaccessible public services combine to become even larger, even more powerful and even more inaccessible?
• Or will greater partnership working prompt current organisations and professions to be more responsive to the needs and desires of service users, help them to reflect on the strengths and limitations of what they currently do, and enable them to challenge established practice where it does not function in the best interests of people who use services?

At the present moment, the jury remains out on both these options, and it is very much up to current practitioners, managers, professions and organisations as to what kind of future they want for themselves and the people they work with.

Do partnerships lead to better outcomes?

Underneath much of the analysis that runs throughout this book are several unanswered questions about the extent to which partnerships lead to better outcomes, how we would know if they did and whether the effort involved in developing partnerships is really worth it. While this is examined in more detail by Dickinson's book in the current series (*Evaluating outcomes in health and social care*), Chapters 1 and 2 of this book have started to develop and reiterate two key points:

- the assumption that partnerships lead to better outcomes is at best unproven, and much existing partnership working remains essentially faith-based;
- both policy makers and frontline services need to focus more on the outcomes they are trying to achieve, before considering the structures and the processes they want to develop as a result.

With this in mind, Chapter 4 now moves on to provide some conceptual frameworks to help explore these issues in more detail, to help develop more locally appropriate approaches to partnership working, and to focus on ensuring that subsequent interagency relationships are more tailored to local contexts and focused on desired outcomes.

Reflective exercises

1. Reflecting on current partnerships, why are you working with current partners? Is it because you want to do this in order to enrich what you currently do? Is it because you recognise that it is in the interests of people who use services? Is it because local or national policy makes you do it? Is it some sort of combination of all of these? With this in mind, what is the best way of encouraging greater partnership working, and how should policy makers and local managers best balance 'carrots' and 'sticks' in order to support the creation of more effective partnerships?

2. Reflecting on your local area, identify two or three key social problems that local partners are trying to resolve. For each of these, who do you need to work with in order to respond best to the issue at stake and do you have the right kind of relationships with relevant partners? If not, what opportunities exist to develop links with such partners?

3. In partnerships where there is significant risk or financial investment involved, are there appropriate safeguards in place

to make sure that all partners feel comfortable with local arrangements and are adequately protected if something goes wrong? In a situation where trust and flexibility are all important, how do you strike the right balance between appropriate risk taking and protection, and between innovation and safe use of taxpayers' money?

4. Where responsibilities and services are delegated to a partner agency, what mechanisms exist to ensure that the partner is delivering on joint commitments? What role should your organisation continue to play in this area, and how can you balance the need to hold your partner to account while at the same time supporting them to deliver mutually beneficial outcomes?

5. Are current partnerships more or less responsive to the needs and wishes of people who use services than previous single agency ways of working? Meeting with a colleague from a different organisational or professional background, discuss the strengths and limitations of current approaches to involving and listening to service users – what scope is there to learn from the best of both approaches in a partnership setting, and what practical steps can you take to contribute to such a change?

6. Reflecting on previous partnerships, did they achieve stated aims? If not, why not? What approaches should current and future partnerships adopt as a result of this learning to ensure that they really do add value and deliver on shared outcomes?

Further reading and resources

This chapter has covered a broad range of issues, and readers may want to follow up specific topics in more detail. As a result, the further reading and resources below are necessarily diverse to enable people to explore all the issues that are relevant to them and their local context.

For more information on delayed hospital discharge, see www. dh.gov.uk and/or www.changeagentteam.org.uk, as well as:

- CSCI's (2004, 2005) studies of reimbursement
- Glasby's (2003) *Hospital discharge*
- Henwood's (2004, 2006) summaries and critique of the new policy

For further discussion of the way in which different approaches to policy making can help to encourage changes in frontline services (or not), see books by Hill (2004), Buse et al (2005) and Baggott (2007).

For material on working with broader partners, see Hudson's (2004) discussion paper on *Whole systems working*, which is available to download free of charge from the Integrated Care Network (www. integratedcarenetwork.gov.uk).

For a discussion of the balance to be struck between effective partnership and local democratic processes, see Skelcher et al's (2004) work on governance and accountability. In particular, their Governance Assessment Tool provides a useful and accessible means of assessing the extent to which partnerships conform to current good practice standards around issues such as accessibility, transparency, accountability and probity.

For examples of what can happen when things go wrong, journalistic accounts of breakdowns in local partnerships can be a helpful resource (see, for example, Batty, 2003; O'Hara, 2006). The Audit Commission (2005) also provides an important discussion of issues of risk, accountability and governance, while official reports such as the investigation into allegations of abuse in a Cornish 'partnership' trust (Healthcare Commission/CSCI, 2006) are important case study material.

—

An accessible discussion of interagency partnerships and governance – *We have to stop meeting like this* – is written by Glasby and Peck (2006), and can be downloaded free of charge from the Integrated Care Network (www.integratedcarenetwork.gov.uk).

4

Useful frameworks and concepts

So far, previous chapters in this book have tended to problematise the concept of partnership working, to critique current policy and practice, and to provide more questions than answers. In some respects, this final substantive chapter is little different in that the issues at stake are so difficult that definitive answers are unlikely to materialise. However, with this caveat in mind, this final substantive chapter seeks to develop previous discussion by summarising a series of useful theoretical frameworks and approaches to help unpick some of the themes and issues cited earlier.

The central importance of outcomes

Above all, almost every previous discussion has returned to the central importance of being clear (with each other, with staff and with service users) what outcomes our partnerships are designed to achieve. This has included:

- a critique of the literature for focusing on issues of process (how well are we working together?) rather than on outcomes (does it make any difference for people who use services?);
- a critique of the tendency to assume that partnership working is a 'good thing' (that leads to better services and hence to better outcomes);
- a critique of the tendency to focus on potentially positive outcomes without necessarily considering the negatives of partnership working;
- a critique of traditional notions of evidence-based practice (which have often been too narrow and too focused on particular types of

research methodology to help us fully understand the relationship between partnerships and outcomes);

- a critique of the tendency to see partnership working as an end in itself rather than as a means to an end;
- a critique of a potential lack of clarity about exactly which forms of partnership may be most appropriate to deliver desired outcomes (see below for further discussion).

Against this background, a useful approach for guarding against these dangers derives from the broader academic literature on 'theories of change' and on 'realistic evaluation'. While these approaches are described in more detail elsewhere, for those interested in following this up (see, for example, Pawson and Tilley, 1997; Connell and Kubisch, 1998; Dickinson, 2006), the Health Services Management Centre (HSMC) tends to use some of the underlying concepts from these approaches in its policy advice and consultancy work. In particular, Figure 4.1 sets out a very simple three-step approach that asks frontline services and practitioners to consider:

- what they are trying to achieve for local people (outcomes)
- how well (or otherwise) current services do this already (context)
- the structures they need to develop as a result (process).

Figure 4.1: Focusing on outcomes

While this is inevitably an over-simplification of a much more complex reality, thinking of partnership working in these terms can be a helpful way of 'seeing the wood for the trees'. Depending on the outcomes concerned, local partners may well decide that they do need some form of partnership, but this is not automatically assumed, and the form of partnership required depends very much on where local services are starting and what they want to achieve. Simple though this may appear, remaining focused on outcomes is extremely difficult in current public services, as many policy makers, managers and practitioners tend to find it easier to think in terms of structures and processes rather than outcomes. This seems to be the result of a series of interrelated issues – the historical legacy that current services have inherited, the tendency for current performance management systems to focus more on process than on outcomes, and the fact that many frontline practitioners are often never asked to think about what they are there to achieve on behalf of the people they serve. In addition, the process of determining outcomes may not be simple and can reveal that different stakeholders have quite different perceptions about what the partnership does/should do. If such an exercise does indeed reveal significant differences, it may well help to explain why partnership working may have been problematic – because different people had very different expectations of the relationship. However, with all these caveats, the fact remains that such an approach can help potential partners to retain a focus on partnership working as a means to an end, rather than as an end in itself (for an example of what can happen when a focus on outcomes is lost, see Box 4.1).

Box 4.1: Remaining focused on outcomes

When asked to focus on outcomes, most public service managers and practitioners quickly drift back into issues of process. Having conducted consultancy and development work around the country, many health and social care communities start to articulate desired outcomes for service users in terms of 'a single point of entry', 'quicker access to services' or 'a single assessment'.

Important though all these things may be, none are outcomes for service users. On the contrary, all are processes, and further facilitation is often needed to help participants understand what kind of outcomes (fewer admissions to hospital, greater life expectancy, greater satisfaction with services etc) they think these processes may help them achieve.

Although this may seem pedantic, being clear about the difference between the overall outcome and the processes that may help you get there is important – we are so conditioned to think about the world in particular ways that we rarely stop to ask ourselves deeper questions about the best way forward. For example, if we really are trying to reduce hospital admissions, a single assessment and a single point of entry may be the right way forward; equally, if this is genuinely what we are trying to achieve then we might do something else entirely (which may or may not involve a partnership).

In an informative if depressing example, one health and social care community was adamant that the outcome it was trying to achieve for local older people was an integrated management team. We are yet to meet any older people who need or want an integrated management team from their health and social care services – this is simply a process that may or may not be the best way of trying to achieve different and better outcomes for people who use services.

Against this background, the remainder of this chapter seeks to explore each stage of the diagram in Figure 4.1, summarising some of the key frameworks and concepts that may help to develop our ability to understand issues of outcome, context and process in more detail.

When seeking to make a clear statement about the outcomes that any given partnership is designed to achieve, recent policy and practice reveals a number of helpful hints. In particular, anecdotal evidence from recent reforms in children's services suggests that this can be most powerful when outcomes are focused on potential benefits for people who use services, when they are expressed positively (that is, 'keeping children safe and well' rather than 'preventing abuse'), and when they are simple and easy to communicate to staff, service users and the public alike. In addition, it is our belief that it is at the stage of articulating desired outcomes that user and carer involvement is most important. All too often, in our experience, services consulting about future provision tend to ask service users for their views on issues of structure or process (and the public consultations that accompanied the transition from primary care groups [PCGs] to PCTs are perhaps an example of this). While users may have a view on health and social services structures, we believe that their input is crucial from day one, and that they should be centrally involved in discussions about desired outcomes – what do they want their lives to be like and how can services support this? After this, involvement in critiquing the current context is also important (in order to establish the extent to which current services deliver user aspirations) – but involvement in what sort of structure is needed as a result is much more technical and much less relevant to many service users. As an example of such an approach, Box 4.2 summarises HSMC's Partnership Outcomes Evaluation Toolkit (POET) as a possible way of approaching this issue (see also the book by Helen Dickinson in this series for further details: *Evaluating outcomes in health and social care*; for further discussion of outcomes more generally see Glendinning et al, 2006).

Box 4.2: The POET approach

The Partnership Outcomes Evaluation Toolkit (POET) is a resource developed by HSMC in order to assist health and social care partnerships to evaluate their work. This web-based resource recognises the importance of both process (that is, how well do partners work together?) and outcome (that is, does the partnership make any difference to those who use services?).

As a result, POET takes a two-pronged approach:

- inviting all staff members to complete an online survey that analyses how the partnership 'feels' to them and also surfacing all the underpinning assumptions about what the partnership is aiming to achieve in terms of outcomes for service users;
- using the information from the staff survey, a research schedule is designed that checks out with service users and carers whether these are the 'right' outcomes to be aiming for and the degree to which the partnership has been successful in changing these outcomes.

In this way, POET is both:

- *formative:* it seeks to evaluate how well partners are working together, helps people to understand and make sense of their current context, and highlights both areas for celebration within the partnership as well as areas where development work is needed;
- *summative:* POET is evaluative in that it requires partnerships to be explicit about desired outcomes and then analyses the degree to which the partnership is successful in achieving these aims.

In compiling a list of desired outcomes, it is also important to consider the *type* of outcomes that the partnership is trying to achieve. Typically, many partnerships have (both stated and unstated) outcomes that focus on benefits to service users (better services), benefits for staff (a richer, more satisfying environment) and benefits for the organisation (better use of scarce resources). Perhaps it is this promise of a potential 'win-win' situation that makes partnership such a tempting concept. However, in considering which type of outcome is being sought, it is important to be open and honest. The danger with some partnerships is that they are seeking economic benefits for partners, but dress this up in the language of service user benefits, and this quickly leads to cynicism and disengagement (particularly for service users who typically see straight through such claims). To aid this process, Mackintosh (1992) provides a helpful distinction between three different types of outcome that a partnership may be trying to achieve:

- *synergy*, bringing together partners with different assets and powers to create something where the whole is greater than the sum of its parts);
- *transformation*, bringing partners together to change the objectives and culture of one or both of the organisations, with the direction of change depending on the power of each individual partner;

- *budget enlargement*, coming together to try to obtain a financial contribution from a third party.

These concepts have since been further developed by Hastings (1996), who provides the typologies set out in Tables 4.1 and 4.2. According to this analysis, Mackintosh's concept of 'synergy' can have a double meaning, referring either to the added value from bringing together and coordinating the resources spent by two or more partners ('resource synergy') or to the new perspectives and innovative solutions that can be created when partners with different cultures and perspectives come together ('policy synergy'). Using these categories, perhaps one of the reasons why partnerships sometimes seem to fail to deliver ambitious aspirations is that service users are seeking the benefits of 'policy synergy', while managers are seeking 'resource synergy'. Or perhaps, as Dickinson et al (2007) illustrate in the case of a care trust, while searching for the benefits of 'policy synergy', partnerships may become too concerned with maintaining the rhetoric of peaceful partnership relationships and so inadvertently stifle potentially more innovative approaches in the name of continuity.

In addition, Hastings (1996) also develops Mackintosh's concept of 'transformation', arguing that different things can happen depending on the power balance. Where power is unequal, this can lead to 'uni-directional transformation' (whereby a more powerful partner tries to change the other to become more like itself and where the reluctant,

Table 4.1: Hastings' (1996) definitions of resource and policy synergy

	Process	Outcome/benefit
Resource synergy	Cooperation and coordination over the spending of resources	Added value from the resources spent: increased effectiveness or efficiency
Policy synergy	Joint approach developed through combining the different perspectives of each partner	New perspectives/ innovative solutions created

Table 4.2: Hastings' (1996) definitions of transformation

	Process	Result
Uni-directional transformation	One or more partners struggle to modify or to change another partner in their own image. Partners do not accept the need to change themselves	One or more partners change their organisational culture or objectives to become more similar to those of another partner. The transforming partner retains its original style or objectives
Mutual transformation	Reciprocal challenges made to the pre-existing culture and objectives of partners, who seek to learn as well as aspire to teach	All partners involved in the process change to some extent. New sets of objectives, operational styles are developed. Differences between partners are reduced

weaker partner is changed against its will). Where both partners accept the need for change and to learn from each other, however, there is the prospect of 'mutual transformation' (whereby all partners change and differences between them begin to reduce).

Understanding what is possible in the current context

While Chapter 2 summarised some of the key frameworks for exploring the current context and the extent of 'partnership readiness', other theoretical approaches and concepts are also useful when trying to (jointly) understand what is desirable and feasible in the current context. In particular, the literature suggests that it is important to be honest and open about the extent to which different partners are genuinely committed to the outcomes in question (as well as about any pressures that may prevent them from prioritising these issues as much as they would like). Without this, there is a danger that partners sign up enthusiastically to desired outcomes that they will never be able to prioritise in practice and that the outcomes at stake are not really important enough to all partners to ensure that the necessary action actually materialises. When this happens, it is easy for trust to erode and for faith in the concept of partnership to reduce. To guard against these dangers, the private sector literature emphasises the importance of focusing partnerships on areas that are of importance to both partners (in the case of the private sector, this often focuses on the supplier and the buyer), with successful outcomes much less likely if the partnership is focusing on something that is important to only one partner and not the other. Where an issue is not strategically important to both parties, then a contractual relationship may be a better way forward. As a simple illustration, Figure 4.2 provides a brief summary of this approach, and this may be helpful for potential partners to use when analysing and developing both current and future relationships.

At the same time, attempts to explore the current context can benefit from an understanding of the different theoretical approaches to interagency working. While this can be extremely complex, a helpful summary is provided by Sullivan and Skelcher (2002), who distinguish between optimist, pessimist and realist approaches. As Table 4.3 suggests,

Figure 4.2: Buyer–supplier strategic perceptions grid

Source: Adapted from Larsson and Bowen (1989, p 221)

—

79

Table 4.3: Optimist, pessimist and realist approaches to partnership working

	Optimist	Pessimist	Realist
Why collaboration happens?	Achieving shared vision	Maintaining/ enhancing position	Responding to new environments
Key assumptions about other partners	Altruistic	Seeking personal or organisational gain	Realise need to change as society changes
Key factors at work	Role of charismatic leaders/ boundary spanners	Power of individual partners and desire for survival	Ability to adapt to changing environment

Source: Adapted from Sullivan and Skelcher (2002)

optimist approaches tend to assume that partnerships occur through a desire to achieve a shared vision, that collaboration will result in positive outcomes for the system as a whole and that partners share a level of altruism. In contrast, pessimist approaches see partnership working as a means for one organisation to enhance their power and resources at the expense of another. In particular, this pursuit of individual or organisational gain can be focused on achieving a solution that helps the one agency deliver its goals, maintains its power and status, maintains or increases its resources and promotes the agency's view of the world and way of doing things. Finally, a realist perspective concentrates more on the wider environment, and sees partnership working as a response to wider political, economic and social factors. As society changes, it is argued, so too must public services. In a fast-moving political and economic context and when faced with a growth in technology and changing public expectations, collaboration is increasingly likely as services seek to respond to developments in the world around them. As a result, the extent to which partnership will be possible in any given situation may well depend on the mix of motives at work in

—

individual partner agencies and on the extent to which it is possible to harness these different approaches in pursuit of shared and mutually beneficial outcomes.

Also useful as a means of understanding the current context is a framework for whole systems working initially proposed by Benson (1975) and explored within the context of children's services by Hudson (2004). For Benson, whole systems working depends on the ability to achieve a degree of balance across eight key areas (see Box 4.3). Applying these in practice, Hudson then demonstrates how this approach can be a useful tool for conducting a 'health check' on the local whole system, helping to understand the local context in more detail and reflect jointly on what is feasible within the current context.

Box 4.3: Benson's (1975) framework for understanding whole systems working

For Benson, it is important to strike a balance between eight different components of the whole system:

- *Domain consensus:* the extent to which there is agreement about the role and scope of each agency's contribution.
- *Ideological consensus:* the extent to which there is agreement regarding the nature of the tasks facing the partnership.
- *Positive evaluation:* the extent to which partners have a positive view of each other.
- *Work coordination:* the extent to which individual partners are prepared to align working patterns.
- *Fulfilment of programme requirements:* the degree of compatibility between the goals of the partnership and the goals of individual agencies.
- *Maintenance of a clear domain of high social importance:* the extent to which there is support for the objectives of the partnership from those affected.
- *Maintenance of resource flows:* the extent to which there is adequate funding for the objectives of the partnership.

- *Defence of the organisational paradigm:* the extent to which partners see themselves as working for the partnership rather than representing their constituency.

Source: Benson (1975), summarised in Hudson (2004, p 9)

How do we get from where we are now to where we want to be?

Once potential partners understand and are clear with each other about what they want to achieve together and about where they are now, the bit in between – what do we do? – ought to be a lot less controversial than is often the case. However, even where partners have used the approach in Figure 4.1 to explore the context and desired outcomes together, it is nearly always issues of structure and process (the 'what do we do?') that generates the most potential tension. When this happens, some of the frameworks and concepts in this final section may help to explore the type of relationship and subsequent partnership arrangements that are needed.

In a classic article on 'the five laws of integration', Leutz (1999) argues that health and social care services may need to work together in different ways depending on what they are trying to achieve. This includes three different levels of integration:

- *Linkage:* appropriate for people with mild, moderate or new needs, linkage involves everyone being clear what services exist and how to access them, so that support is provided by autonomous organisations, but systematically linked.
- *Coordination:* with more explicit structures in place, coordination involves being aware of points of tension, confusion and discontinuity in the system and devising policies and procedures for addressing these.
- *Full integration:* for people with complex or unpredictable needs, full integration involves the creation of new services and approaches with a single approach and pooled funding.

In a similar approach, Peck (2002) and Glasby (2005, 2007) challenge partners to consider the balance they need to strike between depth and breadth of relationship in order to achieve desired outcomes (see Figure 4.3). In any given health and social care community, there will be a range of interagency relationships in different places in this matrix, and potential partners may well find it useful to consider what type of relationship they think they need in order to deliver their joint aspirations. Put another way, this framework encourages local organisations to ask themselves a key question about any given piece of interagency working: 'partnership working with whom and for what'?

Having explored the depth and breadth of relationship needed to achieve desired outcomes, partners should also consider the different structures and processes they could adopt to make their new partnership arrangements as successful as possible. A helpful contribution is made here by research conducted as part of the national evaluation of LSPs (ODPM, 2005b; see also Glasby and Peck, 2006), which sets out some

Figure 4.3: Depth versus breadth of relationship

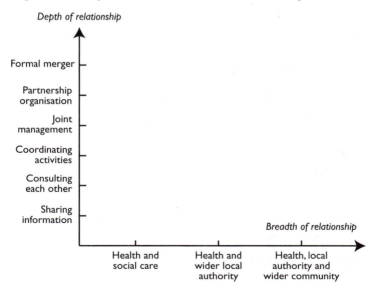

of the different options with regard to modes of governance, approaches to leadership and levels of engagement from partner agencies (see Boxes 4.4 to 4.6). While these frameworks offer little by way of answer to some of the complexities surrounding partnership working, they do provide a useful way of categorising different approaches and circumstances so that potential partners can explore together what kind of relationship they want and how best to organise their subsequent partnership structures. Thus, key questions might include:

- What is the role of the partnership board, and are all partners clear about its primary function (see Box 4.4)?
- What is the role of the chair or lead agency, and how can they best balance the different approaches needed in different situations (see Box 4.5)?
- What levels of engagement are there around the table, and what balance needs to be struck in order for the partnership to deliver its desired outcomes (see Box 4.6)?

Box 4.4: Different modes of governance

- *Advisory:* the board acts as a consultation and discussion forum and often forms the basis for consensus building. It draws its accountability and legitimacy from member organisations, but has no independent power to act.
- *Commissioning:* the partnership has its own staff and authority, is able to implement decisions and commission projects, and therefore has to create its own forms of accountability and legitimacy.
- *Laboratory:* the prime focus is on generating new ideas and new ways of designing local services, drawing on the combined thinking of key stakeholders.
- *Community empowerment:* attention is focused on creating strong networks within the community rather than on the key public agencies.

Source: ODPM (2005b)

Box 4.5: Different approaches to leadership

- *Holding the chair:* setting agendas, managing the business, working the board towards decisions, ensuring that all stakeholders can express their views.
- *Committing partners:* generating collective ownership of and commitment to the partnership from key leaders in partner organisations, establishing accountability to the partnership through influence.
- *Role modelling:* behaving as if joint working matters, respecting diversity, modelling collaboration.
- *Representation:* taking partnership business back into one's own organisation and ensuring that others provide back-up and that the organisation fulfils the partnership's expectations of it.

Source: ODPM (2005b)

Box 4.6: Different levels of engagement

- *Defensive participation:* often new to partnership working, such organisations are concerned about the perceived resource implications or threat of participation – their presence is often defensive (to ensure that their agency does not 'lose out').
- *Opportunistic participation:* such organisations may not see the partnership as core to their own objectives, but are able to see and grasp potential benefits opportunistically. This type of partner is often seen as taking more from the partnership than it contributes.
- *Active participation:* such organisations are strongly committed to the partnership and see taking part as a natural extension of their repertoire for tackling items on their own agenda, as well as those of other partners.

Source: ODPM (2005b)

Overall, this chapter has sought to provide an overview of some key approaches and frameworks that may help to explore the scope for joint working and to design partnership arrangements that help to deliver desired outcomes. Central to this process is the discipline to ignore the temptation to leap straight into debates about structure and about process. Partnerships (and other ways of organising services) are only ever a means to an end, and service users, practitioners, managers, policy makers and researchers all have a duty to make sure that they never become an end in themselves.

Reflective exercises

1. Choose a case study partnership that you have read about, that exists in your local area or that you are working with. Using the context-process-outcome framework in Figure 4.1 above, is it clear (to all partners involved) what the partnership is trying to achieve, how well single agency approaches were performing against these aspirations and why the subsequent partnership has been designed the way it has? When you apply this approach, what chances of success does the partnership have and are there other (potentially unstated) reasons why services may have been designed in this way (above and beyond the formal outcomes of the partnership)?

2. Focusing on another case study partnership, what outcomes does it claim to be trying to achieve? Use the Hastings frameworks in Tables 4.1 and 4.2 to categorise and clarify the type of outcome that the partnership is seeking.

3. Using the framework in Figure 4.2, how important are stated outcomes to each partner, and what chances of success does the partnership have as a result?

4. Reflecting on the possible motives of the different partners involved, to what extent is it possible to see elements of

---

the optimist, pessimist and realist approaches set out in Table 4.3?

5. Using Leutz's categories of linkage, coordination and full integration and/or Peck's model of depth versus breadth, map local partnerships. To what extent do local partners have the right level of relationship with the right organisations in order to achieve desired outcomes?

6. Using the concepts from Boxes 4.4 to 4.6, what role is the partnership board adopting, what leadership approach is it displaying and what balance of engagement does the partnership have?

Further reading and resources

Many of the key texts for this chapter are summarised in the relevant sections above for readers to explore in more depth as appropriate. However:

- for a summary of key theoretical approaches to partnership working, see Sullivan and Skelcher's (2002) *Working across boundaries*
- for more detail on broader theoretical approaches to evaluating complex policy initiatives, see Pawson and Tilley (1997), Connell and Kubisch (1998) and Dickinson (2006)
- for further discussion of whole systems working, see Hudson (2004)

5

Recommendations for policy and practice

Ultimately, the questions, summaries and frameworks set out in this book lead us to make a series of practical recommendations and potential warnings, both for policy and for practice.

For policy makers:

- When seeking to change behaviour in frontline practice, policy makers should resist the temptation to resort to structural change and should not over-estimate the contribution of the power of ideas. Instead, policy should seek to change the accountability of local services and practitioners (both to each other and to people who use services).

- With this in mind, joint targets that hold all relevant local agencies to account for outcomes across the whole system (not just in individual partner agencies) would send an important message about the importance of partnership working.

- The role of government may well be to work with service users and other relevant stakeholders to develop and articulate desired outcomes. Once this is done, it should be the responsibility of local partners to decide how best to organise their interagency relationships in order to achieve such outcomes.

- When seeking to compel the creation of a partnership, it is important to blend elements of hierarchy, market and network in order to maximise the chances of success.

- Greater research is required to understand the extent to which partnerships really do lead to better outcomes (and, if so, what kinds of partnership, for whom and under what circumstances).

- While the current emphasis on evidence-based practice is welcome, this needs to be broadened so that we also learn from 'what does not work', so that we learn from current policy/practice and so that we view service user experiences and practitioner wisdom as potentially valid sources of evidence.

For local organisations and frontline services:

- There is a need to be clearer in our use of language so that terms such as 'partnership working' are used more precisely and so that all local partners have the same understanding of what is being proposed.

- Local partners need to focus first on desired outcomes, before moving on to consider the current context. Issues of process and structure (the 'what do we do?') should come last (and only when we have a jointly agreed understanding of where we are now and where we are trying to get to).

- While some form of partnership may be the best way forward, this is not automatically the case, and a more critical approach to partnership working may well be healthy.

- When asked to work in partnership, always consider who you need to work with and how in order to achieve desired outcomes.

- When designing local partnership arrangements, it is important to reflect carefully on the type of partnership you need, the prime roles it will need to fulfil, the type of leadership it needs and the motives/levels of engagement of key partners.

- While it can sometimes be helpful to be ambitious in scope, it can also be necessary to consider what is feasible in the current context.

Above all, we believe that partnership is an important concept that is probably here to stay. For all the problems and the confusion

—

that partnership working (both the term and the practice) entails, single agency approaches are often insufficient to respond to the complexity of need that public services increasingly face. While we still know relatively little about the impact of partnership working, we are constantly learning more from policy and practice, from the experiences of service users and frontline workers, and from formal research. Provided that we stay focused on the outcomes that interagency working is meant to achieve, partnerships remain a potentially useful means to an end – not the only approach, not an end in themselves, but an extra and important tool in the box when it comes to trying to achieve something different and better for people who use services.

References

6, P., Leat, D., Seltzer, K. and Stoker, G. (2002) *Towards holistic governance*, Basingstoke: Palgrave.

6, P., Goodwin, N., Peck, E. and Freeman, T. (2006) *Managing networks of twenty-first century organisations*, Basingstoke: Palgrave.

Audit Commission (1998) *A fruitful partnership: Effective partnership working*, London: Audit Commission.

Audit Commission (2002) *Integrated services for older people*, London: Audit Commission.

Audit Commission (2005) *Governing partnerships: Bridging the accountability gap*, London: Audit Commission.

Baggott, R. (2007) *Understanding health policy*, Bristol: The Policy Press.

Balloch, S. and Taylor, M. (eds) (2001) *Partnership working: Policy and practice*, Bristol: The Policy Press.

Banks, P. (2002) *Partnerships under pressure: A commentary on progress in partnership working between the NHS and local government*, London: King's Fund.

Barnes, M., Bauld, L., Benzeval, M., Judge, K., Mackenzie, M. and Sullivan, H. (2005) *Health Action Zones: Partnerships for equity*, London: Routledge.

Barrett, G., Sellman, D. and Thomas, J. (eds) (2005) *Interprofessional working in health and social care*, Basingstoke: Palgrave.

Barton, P., Bryan, S. and Glasby, J. et al (2006) *A national evaluation of the costs and outcomes of intermediate care for older people*, Birmingham/ Leicester: Health Services Management Centre and Leicester Nuffield Research Unit.

Batty, D. (2003) 'The end of the affair: row over strategy splits joint management partnership', *The Guardian*, 3 September (www.politics. guardian.co.uk, accessed 20/04/2007).

BBC (2003) 'Trusts to take over child care', 28 January (www.bbc. co.uk, accessed 19/02/2007).

BBC (2005) '"Home alone" deaths for thousands', 29 December (www. bbc.co.uk, accessed 16/02/2007).

Benson, J.K. (1975) 'The inter-organisational network as a political economy', *Administrative Science Quarterly*, vol 20, pp 229-49.

Britnell, M. (2007) 'A freedom framework will unite former foes', *Health Service Journal*, 1 February, pp 18-19.

Burstow, P. (2005) *Dying alone: Assessing isolation, loneliness and poverty* (www.paulburstow.org.uk, accessed 16/02/2007).

Buse, K., Mays, N. and Walt, G. (2005) *Making health policy*, Maidenhead: Open University Press.

Cameron, A. and Lart, R. (2003) 'Factors promoting and obstacles hindering joint working: a systematic review of the research evidence', *Journal of Integrated Care*, vol 11, issue 2, pp 9-17.

Carpenter, J. and Dickinson, H. (2008) *Interprofessional education and training*, Bristol: The Policy Press.

CHI (Commission for Health Improvement) (2003) *Investigation into matters arising from care on Rowan Ward, Manchester Mental Health and Social Care Trust*, London: CHI (now Healthcare Commission).

Connell, J.P. and Kubisch, A.C. (1998) 'Applying a theory of change approach to the evaluation of comprehensive community initiatives: progress, prospects and problems', in K. Fulbright-Anderson, A.C. Kubisch, and J.P. Connell (eds) *New approaches to evaluating community initiatives: Volume 2 – Theory, measurement and analysis*, Washington, DC: The Aspen Institute.

Coopers & Lybrand (1993) *Making a success of acquisitions*, London: Coopers & Lybrand.

Craig, G. and Manthorpe, J. (1999) *Unfinished business? Local government reorganisation and social services*, Bristol: The Policy Press in association with the Joseph Rowntree Foundation.

CSCI (Commission for Social Care Inspection) (2004) *Leaving hospital – The price of delays*, London: CSCI.

CSCI (2005) *Leaving hospital – Revisited*, London: CSCI.

DH (Department of Health) (1998) *Partnership in action: New opportunities for joint working between health and social services – A discussion document*, London: DH.

DH (2000) *The NHS Plan: A plan for investment, a plan for reform*, London: The Stationery Office.

DH (2001) *Valuing People: A new strategy for learning disability for the 21st century*, London: The Stationery Office.

DH (2006) *Our health, our care, our say*, London: The Stationery Office.

Dickinson, H. (2006) 'The evaluation of health and social care partnerships: an analysis of approaches and synthesis for the future', *Health and Social Care in the Community*, vol 14, no 5, pp 375-83.

Dickinson, H. (2008) *Evaluating outcomes in health and social care*, Bristol: The Policy Press.

Dickinson, H. and Glasby, J. (eds) (forthcoming: 2008) *Partnership working in health and social care: Some international perspectives*, Oxford: Blackwell.

Dickinson, H., Peck, E. and Davidson, D. (2007) 'Opportunity seized or missed? A case study of leadership and organisational change in the creation of a care trust', *Journal of Interprofessional Care*, vol 21, no 5, pp 503-13.

Dickinson, H., Peck, E. and Smith, J. (2006) *Leadership in organisational transition – What can we learn from research evidence? Summary report*, Birmingham: Health Services Management Centre.

Dowling, B., Powell, M. and Glendinning, C. (2004) 'Conceptualising successful partnerships', *Health and Social Care in the Community*, vol 12, no 4, pp 309-17.

Edwards, A., Barnes, M. and Plewis, I. et al (2006) *Working to prevent the social exclusion of children and young people: Final lessons from the national evaluation of the Children's Fund*, Birmingham: Department for Education and Skills, University of Birmingham.

Field, J. and Peck, E. (2003) 'Mergers and acquisitions in the private sector: what are the lessons for health and social services?', *Social Policy and Administration*, vol 37, no 7, pp 742-55.

Fraser, D. (2003) *The evolution of the British welfare state* (3rd edn), Basingstoke: Palgrave.

Fulop, N., Protopsaltis, G., King, A., Allen, P., Hutchings, A. and Normand, C. (2005) 'Changing organisations: a study of the context and processes of mergers of health care providers in England', *Social Science and Medicine*, vol 60, no 1, pp 119-30.

Fulop, N., Protopsaltis, G., Hutchings, A., King, A., Allen, P., Normand, C. and Walters, R. (2002) 'Process and impact of mergers of NHS trust: multicentre case study and management cost analysis', *British Medical Journal*, vol 325, pp 246-52.

Glasby, J. (2003) *Hospital discharge: Integrating health and social care*, Abingdon: Radcliffe Medical Press.

Glasby, J. (2004) *Working together to meet the needs of people with learning disabilities: A report of a national workshop*, Birmingham: Health Services Management Centre/Valuing People Support Team.

Glasby, J. (2005) 'The integration dilemma: how deep and how broad to go?', *Journal of Integrated Care*, vol 13, no 5, pp 27-30.

Glasby, J. (2007) *Understanding health and social care*, Bristol: The Policy Press.

Glasby, J. and Beresford, P. (2006) 'Who knows best? Evidence-based practice and the service user contribution', *Critical Social Policy*, vol 26, no 1, pp 268-84.

Glasby, J. and Littlechild, R. (2002) *Social work and direct payments*, Bristol: The Policy Press.

Glasby, J. and Littlechild, R. (2004) *The health and social care divide: The experiences of older people* (2nd edn), Bristol: The Policy Press.

Glasby, J. and Peck, E. (eds) (2003) *Care trusts: Partnership working in action*, Abingdon: Radcliffe Medical Press.

Glasby, J. and Peck, E. (2006) *We have to stop meeting like this: The governance of inter-agency partnerships*, Leeds: Integrated Care Network.

Glasby, J., Walshe, K. and Harvey, G. (eds) (2007) 'What counts as "evidence" in "evidence-based practice"?', special edition of *Evidence & Policy*, vol 3, no 3.

Glendinning, C., Powell, M. and Rummery, K. (eds) (2002a) *Partnerships, New Labour and the governance of welfare*, Bristol: The Policy Press.

Glendinning, C., Hudson, B., Hardy, B. and Young, R. (2002b) *National evaluation of notifications for the use of the Section 31 partnership flexibilities in the Health Act 1999: Final project report*, Leeds/Manchester: Nuffield Institute for Health/National Primary Care Research and Development Centre.

Glendinning, C., Clarke, S., Hare, P., Kotchetkova, I., Maddison, J. and Newbronner, L. (2006) *Outcomes-focused services for older people*, London: Social Care Institute for Excellence.

Godfrey, M., Keen, J., Townsend, J. et al (2005) *An evaluation of intermediate care for older people: Final report*, Leeds: University of Leeds.

Greig, R. (2000) 'The locality learning disability service', Paper presented to the Community Care Development Centre/King's College London Conference on 'Community Learning Disability Teams', 13 December, London.

Greig, R. and Poxton, R. (2001) 'From joint commissioning to partnership working – will the new policy framework make a difference?', *Managing Community Care*, vol 9, no 4, pp 32–8.

Hardy, B., Hudson, B. and Waddington, E. (2003) *Assessing strategic partnership: The Partnership Assessment Tool*, London: Office of the Deputy Prime Minister/Nuffield Institute for Health.

Hastings, A. (1996) 'Unravelling the process of "partnership" in urban regeneration policy', *Urban Studies*, vol 33, no 2, pp 253–68.

Healthcare Commission/CSCI (Commission for Social Care Inspection) (2006) *Joint investigation into the provision of services for people with learning disabilities at Cornwall Partnership NHS Trust*, London: Healthcare Commission.

Health Service Journal (2006) 'Government launches media offensive amid £500m deficit', *Health Service Journal*, 8 June, p 5.

Henwood, M. (2004) *Reimbursement and delayed discharges*, Leeds: Integrated Care Network.

Henwood, M. (2006) 'Effective partnership working: a case study of hospital discharge', *Health and Social Care in the Community*, vol 14, no 5, pp 400–7.

Hill, M. (2000) *Understanding social policy* (6th edn), Oxford: Blackwell.

Hill, M. (2004) *The public policy process* (4th edn), Harlow: Pearson Education.

HM Treasury (2003) *Every Child Matters*, London: The Stationery Office.

Hudson, B. (2000) 'Inter-agency collaboration: a sceptical view', in A. Brechin, H. Brown and M.A. Eby (eds) *Critical practice in health and social care*, Milton Keynes: Open University Press.

Hudson, B. (2002) 'Integrated care and structural change in England: the case of care trusts', *Policy Studies*, vol 23, no 2, pp 77-95.

Hudson, B. (2004) *Whole systems working*, Leeds: Integrated Care Network.

Jelphs, K. and Dickinson, H. (2008) *Working in teams*, Bristol: The Policy Press.

Johri, M., Béland, F. and Bergman, H. (2003) 'International experiments in integrated care for the elderly: a synthesis of the evidence', *International Journal of Geriatric Psychiatry*, vol 18, pp 222-35.

Jupp, B. (2000) *Working together: Creating a better environment for cross-sector partnerships*, London: Demos.

Kodner, D. (2006) 'Whole system approaches to health and social care partnerships for the frail elderly: an exploration of North American models and lessons', *Health and Social Care in the Community*, vol 14, no 5, pp 384-90.

Laming, H. (2003) *The Victoria Climbié Inquiry*, London: The Stationery Office.

Larsson, R. and Bowen, D.E. (1989) 'Organization and customer: managing design and coordination of services', *Academy of Management Review*, vol 14, no 2, pp 213-33.

Leathard, A. (ed) (1994) *Going inter-professional: Working together for health and welfare*, Hove: Routledge.

Leichsenring, K. and Alaszewski, A. (eds) (2004) *Providing integrated health and social care for older persons: A European overview of issues at stake*, Aldershot: Ashgate.

Leutz, W. (1999) 'Five laws for integrating medical and social services: lessons from the United States and the United Kingdom', *The Milbank Quarterly*, vol 77, no 1, pp 77-110.

Ling, T. (2000) 'Unpacking partnership: the case of health', in J. Clarke and S.M.E. Gewirtz (eds) *New managerialism, new welfare?*, London: Sage Publications.

McCulloch, A. and Parker, C. (2004) 'Inquiries, assertive outreach and compliance: is there a relationship?', in N. Stanley and J. Manthorpe (eds) *The age of the inquiry: Learning and blaming in health and social care*, London: Routledge.

Mackintosh, M. (1992) 'Partnership: issues of policy and negotiation', *Local Economy*, vol 7, no 3, pp 210-24.

Manthorpe, J., Cornes, M., Rapaport, J., Moriaty, J., Bright, L., Clough, R. and Iliffe, S. (2006) 'Commissioning community well-being: focus on older people and transport', *Journal of Integrated Care*, vol 14, no 4, pp 28-37.

Markwell, S., Watson, J., Speller, V., Platt, S. and Younger, T. (2003) *The Working Partnership*, London: Health Development Agency (now NICE).

Means, R. and Smith, R. (1998) *From Poor Law to community care*, Basingstoke: Macmillan.

Means, R., Richards, S. and Smith, R. (2003) *Community care: Policy and practice* (3rd edn), Basingstoke: Palgrave.

ODPM (Office of the Deputy Prime Minister) (2005a) *A process evaluation of the negotiation of pilot local area agreements*, London: ODPM.

ODPM (2005b) *Evaluation of local strategic partnerships: Interim report*, London: ODPM.

ODPM (2007) *Evidence of savings, improved outcomes, and good practice attributed to local area agreements*, London: ODPM.

ODPM and Department of Transport (2006) *National evaluation of local strategic partnerships: Formative evaluation and action research programme, 2002-2005*, London: ODPM.

O'Hara, M. (2006) 'Pain but no gain', *The Guardian*, 10 May (www.politics.guardian.co.uk, accessed 20/04/2007).

—

O'Keeffe, M., Hills, A., Doyle, M. et al (2007) *UK study of abused and neglect of older people: Prevalence survey report*, London: National Centre for Social Research.

Pawson, R. and Tilley, N. (1997) *Realistic evaluation*, London: Sage Publications.

Payne, M. (2000) *Teamwork in mutliprofessional care*, Basingstoke: Macmillan.

Peck, E. (2002) 'Integrating health and social care', *Managing Community Care*, vol 10, no 3, pp 16-19.

Peck, E. and Dickinson, H. (2008) *Managing and leading in inter-agency settings*, Bristol: The Policy Press.

Peck, E. and Freeman, T. (2005) *Reconfiguring PCTs: Influences and options* (briefing paper prepared for the NHS Alliance), Birmingham: Health Services Management Centre.

Peck, E. and 6, P. (2006) *Beyond delivery: Policy implementation as sense-making and settlement*, Basingstoke: Palgrave Macmillan.

Peck, E., Gulliver, P. and Towell, D. (2002) *Modernising partnerships: Evaluation of Somerset's innovations in the commissioning and organisation of mental health services – Final report*, London: Institute for Applied Health and Social Policy, King's College London.

Powell, M. and Dowling, B. (2006) 'New Labour's partnerships: comparing conceptual models with existing forms', *Social Policy and Society*, vol 5, no 2, pp 305-14.

Rodríguez, C., Langley, A., Béland, F. and Denis, J.-L. (2007) 'Governance, power, and mandated collaboration in an interorganizational network', *Administration and Society*, vol 39, no 2, pp 150-93.

Rummery, K. and Glendinning, C. (2000) *Primary care and social services: Developing new partnerships for older people*, Abingdon: Radcliffe Medical Press.

Rycroft-Malone, J., Seers, K., Titchen, A., Harvey, G., Kitson, A. and McCormack, B. (2004) 'What counts as evidence in evidence-based practice?', *Journal of Advanced Nursing*, vol 47, no 1, pp 81-90.

Skelcher, C., Mathur, N. and Smith, M. (2004) *Effective partnership and good governance: Lessons for policy and practice*, Birmingham: Institute of Local Government Studies, University of Birmingham.

SSI (Social Services Inspectorate)/Audit Commission (2004) *Old virtues, new virtues: An overview of the changes in social care services over the seven years of Joint Reviews in England, 1996-2003*, London: SSI/Audit Commission.

Sullivan, H. and Skelcher, C. (2002) *Working across boundaries: Collaboration in public services*, Basingstoke: Palgrave.

Thomson, A.M. and Perry, J.L. (1998) 'Can AmeriCorps build communities?', *Nonprofit and Voluntary Sector Quarterly*, vol 27, no 4, pp 399-420.

Thompson, G., Frances, J., Levacic, R. and Mitchell, J. (1991) *Markets, hierarchies and networks: The coordination of social life*, London: Sage Publications in association with The Open University.

University of East Anglia (2007) *Children's Trust pathfinders: Innovative partnerships for improving the well-being of children and young people*, Norwich: University of East Anglia in association with the National Children's Bureau.

Walshe, K. (2003) 'Foundation hospitals: a new direction for NHS reform', *Journal of the Royal Society of Medicine*, vol 96, pp 106-10.

Index